THE JOY OF FEELING FIT

THE JOY

photographs by the author

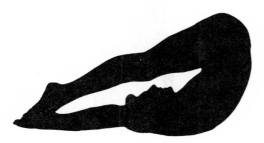

OF FEELING FIT

Nicholas Kounovsky

 E. P. DUTTON & CO., INC. • NEW YORK • 1971

Published simultaneously in Canada by Clarke, Irwin & Company Limited, Toronto and Vancouver

Designed by The Etheredges

To Gally, Vera, Kyra, and Nicky
and with sincere gratitude
to all my friends who helped me
in bringing this book to be

CONTENTS

INTRODUCTION

A stallion galloping in the field, a kitten leaping among fallen leaves, a bird gliding through the air—these actions are expressions of joyful fitness. A gymnast smoothly performing difficult feats, a tennis player executing perfect strokes while covering the entire court, a virtuoso musician enchanting audiences, a swimmer skimming the surface of the water, a pole-vaulter leaping into the air, a couple dancing with lightness and grace—this is harmony of motion, the expression of the joy of feeling free and fit.

Nothing is more beautiful than a well-coordinated body in action. And nothing is more easily attained—if you exercise properly. Because I have been perfecting active bodies for over three decades, I am convinced that anyone can turn into the "better version of himself" he dreams of being.

We are all in search of a mysterious "something else." Many of my students —of all ages, personalities, and styles of life—discover this "something" in the joy of feeling fit. Each one, after a personalized check-up test, has followed a program of progressive training designed to educate, develop, revitalize, and maintain a renewed body in a spirit of joy and relaxation. In the following pages you too will learn how to take full advantage of this most precious gift—your body.

The Joy of Feeling Fit is intended as a fitness manual for the home. It presents not a theory but a practical system based on the factors that activate the human body. Because my conviction is that there are six of these basic factors, the method is called *Sixometry*. Through it exhaustion becomes obsolete, and every action can be made meaningful and productive. The emphasis is on harmonious design and fitness. Even in our sedentary, automated, often unhealthy world, Sixometry works.

Like sports cars or jet planes, we all have sources of energy and basic factors that permit us to perform. If the human machine is to perform at peak capacity, every one of its elements should be in perfect working order. This is best accomplished by specifically directed movements that are called *engineered exercises* or, sometimes, *gymnaks*.

No two people are ever alike—nor should their exercise programs, especially at the beginning, be the same. Regardless of your present shape (physical or mental), you can train and harmonize your body until it is functioning the way it is supposed to function. And you can keep it that way if your fitness program is well designed.

FITNESS À LA CARTE

WHAT IS FITNESS?

Fitness eludes specific definition. It involves everything from emotional strength to perfect balance, from a wonderful figure to an inner peace.

Otrada is a Russian word that describes a happy feeling, a state of enchanting well-being.

Unfortunately, most of us lose this sensation of delight somewhere between childhood and early adolescence. Even children often miss the chance to nourish their bodies and cultivate this joy.

The pace of modern life attacks fitness on all fronts. Human beings are highly adaptable, and once habituated, they survive by a kind of rudimentary physical maintenance: eating, sleeping, tolerating tensions, exerting effort only when absolutely necessary.

Just as all parts of the body are integrated and interdependent, so are all the elements of fitness. If any part of you is below par, whatever you do and however you feel and look is immediately affected, whether you realize it or not.

How many have felt truly fit? Too often people in old age or even in middle age resign themselves unnecessarily to a lack of fitness, a fact I have observed in innumerable cases.

After rediscovering the value of physical activity, a friend recently told me, "I was being so unfair to myself all those years, without even knowing it."

A student of mine who happened to be a doctor said, "My exercising with you has become the most wonderful addiction and, by all means, the healthiest!"

You may easily overlook some of the usual symptoms of lack of fitness: puffing up a flight of stairs, straining to tie a shoelace, or unexpectedly losing balance. But if you have started to refuse invitations you would really like to accept, such as to a tennis game or a dance, your distress is harder to ignore.

Sports, games, dances, and even gymnastic feats are not beyond your grasp —unless you have decided that they are. After beginning even a minimal exercise program, you can actually enjoy renewed physical energy and take pride in fresh skills and fitness.

In using Sixometry, which is derived from engineering principles as well as from knowledge of anatomy and physiology, we divide the movements of the human body into their basic attributes or factors. Once you know which factors to perfect or develop, and understand what you are and how you move, you can tailor the exercises in this book to your special needs.

THE HARMONY OF THE BODY

It is amusing but true that because we are so constantly covered up, we are almost unaware of what is beneath our clothing. Unless a slight bulge shows through, we tend to ignore the areas we can't see, treating our body almost as if it belonged to someone else.

But, however much of it has so far been ignored, it is precisely this body in its totality that you will be exercising. Treat it as you would a violin, a new guitar, a stereo tape deck, or a motorcycle; that is, learn enough about it to tune it up to top performance. Any complex machinery that you understand well yields the greatest returns in use and enjoyment.

Due to great variations in physical proportion, bodily structure, and chemical composition, there are no two identical persons in the world. Even a pair of "identical" twins have bodies that respond in quite individual ways to physical activity.

Weight and size are constant preoccupations. But you should not forget the difference between a massive pound of feathers and a highly compact pound of apples.

BODY DENSITY

Your body may increase in weight by 10 percent (or more) without changing its actual size. Your size can change just as radically without affecting your weight. A weight-conscious friend recently returned from her vacation cruise and exclaimed, "I don't know what happened. I was very careful to keep my weight exactly the same. But I can't fit into any of my clothes." She was mystified that her measurements had increased while the scales still reported her normal weight.

At the same time, her husband's waist had remained a slim 32.

"My clothes still fit me perfectly," he reported. "I behaved myself on our trip." But when the scales showed his weight had increased by several pounds, he was as curious as his wife.

The tricks that seem to have been played here involve nothing more than body density. Because the wife had remained inactive, her muscles had lost their firmness; she ate more than usual and added fat to her body tissues, increasing her size. Because fat is lighter than muscle, however, her weight remained constant. In her husband's case, although he too had eaten more than usual, a great deal of exercise helped him to eliminate unnecessary fat, making his body tissues heavier while he remained the same volume or size.

From this evidence it is obvious that outward appearance does not accurately indicate weight.

The following four points are basic to an understanding of the dynamics of body density:

1. You have low body density if, in your daily movements, you don't use up the food energy that you absorb but instead store it in the form of fatty deposits in your tissues. This increases size more than weight. Individuals with low density have a tendency to be less healthy or even malnourished. Fatty tissues are larger in size than other body tissues and they are lazy in burning energy.

2. You have high body density if you burn up more food energy than you absorb and have to use stored energy as well to keep you going. This converts the fatty contents of your tissues into muscles (or firms them), and thus weight can rise while dimensions remain the same.

3. If you expend the same amount of energy you absorb, you keep a stable body density.
4. Your body density can change.

From personal experience I know that when I am extremely active, my density is very high. I can eat huge meals and increase my weight by as much as 12 pounds while my measurements don't change. I can actually sense the changes in density. When it is at its highest, I can walk on the bottom of a swimming pool, and I need to make a special effort to surface.

Remember, the higher the density, the fitter you are. Fat-free tissues yield more energy and work with less strain. If you want to derive the most from food, which is your fuel, and to achieve the greatest freedom of movement, high density is your goal.

BODY TYPES

People come in all shapes and sizes. To simplify matters, human bodies are commonly divided into three basic types. Each of these is an extreme example, and most of us share the characteristics of one, two, or even all three groups.

Once you determine your predominant type, you will be able to select the exercise procedure that is most appropriate for you. By following the right procedure, you can minimize the undesirable aspects (of figure, posture, etc.) that your type implies and perfect your naturally positive qualities. In other words, it is to your advantage to work according to your type.

The extreme *ectomorph* has relatively little flesh to cover small bones, and is therefore thin. His nervous system often keeps his muscles overtensed, and he tends to use his energy without restraint. Despite a good appetite and the ability to absorb great quantities of food, his body has difficulty building up extra tissues and gaining weight.

The extreme *endomorph* generally has a jovial, relaxed manner; he is protected by soft, even flabby tissues that give him a round, obese appearance. An extra weight load has to be carried by unprepared muscles, and a person of this type may well be taxing his heart.

The extreme *mesomorph* has a square, muscular build, with firm flesh, and is usually vigorous. In fact, the mesomorph has a tendency to overexert himself. He has a high body density, and his flesh is relatively free of excess fat.

While it is certainly beyond your power to change your basic constitution, transform your nervous system, or change the size of your brain, you can minimize undesirable physical characteristics. By following a personal fitness program, you will find that you can change—sometimes radically—your measurements, postural habits, and physical factors.

VIVE LA DIFFÉRENCE

One fact remains inflexible: there is man and there is woman. And as the first step in seeking personal fitness, we must recognize the difference. The two sexes will always strive for unique goals in appearance, physical competence, and quality of movements.

Besides keeping her body supple and her flesh firm, a woman wants to achieve fluent coordination and flawless movements. Any unfeminine movements must be eliminated from her exercise regime. She must also avoid the overdevelopment of visible muscles, while still achieving enough strength and endurance for the tasks of daily life.

Physically, a man must be strong but not brutal, calm but not sluggish; his energies must be enduring, so that he will be stable in orientation, limber and yet sturdy in physical activity, and prudent in behavior.

Time and again I have seen regular and correct physical activity help individuals affirm their personalities and reassert their masculine or feminine nature. In many cases the individuals had not even a slight suspicion that such a reassertion was needed—until they began their program.

The exercise programs outlined in this manual permit both sexes to accentuate their positive qualities and gain the fitness that enhances their sexual identity, their appeal, and their image in a highly sex-oriented world. I also recommend that you encourage your children to join the family fitness programs. They will profit immensely from the engineered exercises of Sixometry.

CHILDREN AND ADOLESCENTS

Children

Man is the only member of the animal kingdom who cannot learn to walk, run, jump, or fly in a matter of hours. During the process of evolution, we seem to have lost our innate physical coordination and sense of orientation. For this reason we should begin to gain them back during early youth.

We tend to assume that children automatically possess supple bodies, excellent endurance, agility, physical competence, and even flat tummies—but this is not always so. Youngsters need thorough physical training and a "Sixometric education" as vitally as adults do.

Children should be fit. They may be short or tall, but they should not be overweight or underweight. Youngsters have individual personalities as well as unique bodies, and they respond well to activities designed for their particular needs: A high-strung child can be helped to relax and move with grace, while a slow-paced youth can gain valuable energy through his exercises.

By observing your child carefully (both physically and psychologically), you can direct his physical activities and supplement his school gym program. Children learn fast and acquire languages and skills rapidly. Your child is a great imitator as well, and he needs only the proper encouragement and guidance to gain confidence and freedom of movement during his growing years.

Adolescents

Young adults on the verge of maturity have always been particularly in need of energetic physical activity. Furthermore it is during these busy years, when they are most distracted by new social and intellectual interests, that they may easily neglect exercise.

At this stage of life, personalities begin to take more permanent form. It is especially important to overcome any signs of shyness, aggressiveness, or nervousness that might threaten an individual's happiness. The right kind of exercise, along with a careful diet, will insure any teen-ager the foundation for lifelong physical fitness.

As children turn into adults, activity should remain a natural part of their lives; they should not refrain from activity for fear of messing up a hairdo or a dress or shirt. Yet often they underestimate the value of physical fitness. But to face the world today one *has* to be fit.

Athletics, sports, games, dances lead to improved fitness. Sports that will be enjoyed for many years—above all, perennial sports like tennis, swimming, skiing and skating—should be encouraged now. The time spent on them will never be regretted.

According to leading authorities, physical middle age comes between twenty and eighty. Your personal physical fitness program may decide when it comes for you.

HOW DO WE FUNCTION?

One reason that the average person knows so little about how he moves is that he seems to function rather well without supervision. We give our automobiles a periodic checkup—the law requires it. But unless he feels something is amiss, the average person assumes that his body is in top working condition. He is probably wrong. Man is a combination of interconnected, simultanous systems that all need frequent adjustment. Through motion, we can actually "tune ourselves up." Once you understand what happens when you move, you will be able to improve yourself through movement.

We are built architecturally, with a skeleton as our structural frame. Our bones are held together principally by ligaments, tendons, and muscles. Most of our joints are mobile, permitting us to perform in countless ways, from beachcombing to walking in space.

We use mechanical principles to move. Our muscles provide us with the forces of motion. Bones become levers and joints serve as pivots.

To move well we constantly alter the rhythm and intensity of our actions and reactions. Some of these motions occur thousands of times each day, usually without our even thinking about them. Others—such as a tennis stroke or a kiss—require more strategy or savoir-faire.

All of these functions are controlled by the (sometimes temperamental) nervous system, which is a kind of electronic center for the body. Nerve impulses travel invisibly through intricate passages, supplying the current that "turns on" muscles and organs and keeps them working correctly.

The body itself is a small but complex chemical laboratory that works night and day. By breathing and eating we are able to feed our tissues with the fuel they need to perform their work of maintaining or building themselves up. Many of these chemical processes are unimaginably complex (muscular action is a process that still baffles medical scientists). There are actually fourteen separate chemical operations involved when you assimilate a single lump of sugar into your system.

YOUR CENTER OF GRAVITY

What do Acapulco's famous rock divers, a juggling tightrope walker, and you (each time you stand up) have in common? Each one demonstrates the startling power of the force of gravity on the human body, and the existence of the body's own center of gravity.

Whenever I mention this vital element to a class, someone will laugh and say, "I don't need to work on my gravity. After all, I'm not falling down, am I?" But as soon as I ask the class members simply to stand on one leg—with their eyes closed—the protests stop. Without periodic practice, one's powers of balance are bound to become slightly rusty.

When you stand and then lean slowly to one side while keeping your body straight, you will find yourself off balance at a certain moment. To save yourself from falling, you then spontaneously bring your body into balance. But what really happens?

You lose your equilibrium the second you reach a specific point that goes beyond your range of control. This point is your body's center of gravity; it is an imaginary spot situated approximately in the center of your body.* Gravitational attraction is constantly acting upon that point, and when you control it, you are in balance.

* The center of the body and hence of gravity is slightly higher in men than in women.

While it is the magic of your muscle fibers that makes you move, it is this sense of equilibrium that helps you move correctly, whether you are in outer space, on earth, or in water. The center of gravity is thus very much like an invisible friend; once you know how to control it, you will be capable of more graceful, coordinated, and effective movements.

Quite often the simple use of the center of gravity is totally ignored. Not long ago a group of instructors at a well-known ice-skating rink in New York admitted the difficulty they were having teaching others to ice skate. While I am not an ice champion myself, I could see that they were forgetting about gravity's pull on the body; once they understood that the center of gravity must be over the skate, they could communicate this to their pupils; the results were exciting to watch.

Another good example is the role that the center of gravity played when I was helping war victims, especially amputation cases, rehabilitate themselves by finding their new balance. They learned faster than when they had been taught by a method of repetition used at that time in hospitals.

To help you understand and improve your handling of the effect of gravity upon your body, you should practice a variety of movements covering 360 degrees, performing them in several different positions. You will gain better control of your body, and you will use less energy as you move, whether you are playing an active sport or performing your daily tasks.

POSTURE AND GAIT

Both thoroughbred horses and a marching procession of political dignitaries display their inner importance by the way they walk. Posture and gait tell the world how you think about yourself. By a change in them a shy girl can turn herself into a high-fashion model, or an insecure man can become a source of strength and confidence for those around him. Control of your walk means control of your attitudes. I have seen the simplest postural corrections make exciting changes in an individual's life, and it can in yours as well.

Your posture is determined by the way you hold each part of your body—from your head to your toes. And this posture may affect your breathing, general health, emotional attitudes, and of course the image you project to the world.

As the bones in your body are held together by ligaments, tendons, and muscles, a specific set of muscles supports each bone in the best postural position. Without muscles your bones would hang down almost vertically. Tonic muscular contractions (which I shall discuss later in this section) provide the tension needed to maintain an ideal position.

Because your body is far more maneuverable than any machine ever built, perfect posture is a highly complex matter. There is a right posture for every single position your body can assume.

Later in this book you will find special exercises for improving posture. Stretching and hanging exercises (suspending from a trapeze or a Nakbar,* for example) will help to relieve dangerous compression on the wrong joints. Once you train the proper muscles, you will easily be able to keep your head up, chest wide, shoulders back, spine straight, abdomen in, hips relaxed, and your entire body well balanced and light on its feet, ready for action.

HOW DO WE MOVE?

How do your muscles work?

You can't even blink an eye without contracting muscle fibers. Every time you move, your body is obeying elementary principles of muscular contraction, the essence of any motion.

When a muscle contracts, whether you feel it or not, it shrinks the distance between its attachments to the bones. Even if the muscle appears to bulge a bit in its effort, it is still actually shortening.

Muscles are composed of groups of thin fibers. The actual contraction is a combination of chemical, electrical, and mechanical reactions; these make the muscle fibers change form, increasing in width and shortening in length—all without changing volume. All muscles respond to stimulation by contracting and then springing back to their original state.

You don't really "stretch" a muscle when you exercise, as is commonly believed. Stretching occurs only when the muscle itself is inactive and is stretched by either an outside force or another, unrelated muscle. A working muscle performs in response to your demands. Holding a package, hanging from a rope by your hands, or holding a basketball, all call for *static* contractions, that is, the muscle does not change its length. A muscle in a static contraction that also opposes a force equal to or greater than its own is in an *isometric* contraction.

For most movements the muscle must change its length. When you lift a heavy load or climb a rope, the muscle shortens and the contraction is called *concentric*. When you lower a weight or descend a rope, your muscles elongate and the contraction is called *eccentric*. And if, as in lifting a weight, the muscle changes length while the resistance to the muscle remains constant, the concentric or eccentric contractions are called *isotonic*.

* For information concerning this and other exercising apparatus, see page 182.

Muscles are always in a state of *tonic* contraction; this is what is meant by "muscle tone."

I have found that quality and response vary greatly among individuals and can be improved with proper exercise. Many factors affect the strength of your muscles—your physical or mental state, whether your muscles are warmed up, and whether various toxins are present in your body. Fear makes you run faster, joy makes you perform better; pride, anger, and anxiety can affect the performance of the most inactive ectomorph or overdeveloped mesomorph.

In a complete fitness program, each muscle should be used completely in each contraction. Whatever action you avoid will become a weak link in your chain of physical activity. Hanging from a rope will not teach you to climb it, and spending time on static contractions alone will not prepare you for a life of lively movement.

The exercise programs in this manual are carefully designed to include every kind of muscular contraction. Eventually you will acquire the same ease in straightening yourself up from a bending position (working the spine in a concentric motion) as you have in bending down (working it in an eccentric motion). Remember too that when your muscles are contracted in one position for too long, they become painfully cramped, as they do when you hold a steering wheel tightly without exercising your fingers periodically. You can avoid such problems by following the engineered sequences of movements in this manual, planning them according to your personal requirements and needs.

PERSONAL PROGRAMMING

EXERCISE DOSAGE AND PROCEDURE

Exercises must be tailored to fit *you* personally so that each move counts. Recently Russia's Olympic coaches personalized their standard athletic training program for the first time. They finally acknowledged that all athletes cannot be trained the same way, not even for the same sport. No two people are exactly alike. A personal regime is more efficient and more fun.

Once you have taken the Sixometric tests and have learned your precise needs, you can direct your exercises at the areas where you are weak. It will be like having a private instructor to guide every stretch-and-bend of your program. You will do only those exercises that you can carry out effectively without strain, and thus you will be insured of immediate as well as long-term success. Such a stimulating prospect is perhaps the greatest incentive for making a personal exercise program part of your daily-life scheme.

One of the most important discoveries of my career has been the amazing variety of ways that there are to exercise and the radical differences in the results. Which exercises you perform, how many, and in what way should be as specifically indicated for you as your physician's prescription.

With over four hundred muscles, your body is capable of performing an enormous variety of motions. The specific movements you select will determine the quality of your exercising. You must also choose the proper rhythm, because the rhythm or pace will soothe or stimulate, relax or invigorate, or may even leave you weary.

The intensity of each exercise is the amount of effort required. This depends on the position of the body in terms of leverage and on the weight or force involved. The intensity must be progressive to be effective.

The number of times each exercise should be performed is still controversial, but without a doubt it is a vital decision. I have found that performing each exercise 6 times provides the best results, except in exercises for endurance and speed.

The order in which the exercises are done and the timing of rest periods are contributing factors toward success or failure. You should not start jogging before a light setting-up session or carry on a long session without pausing for adequate periods of rest to restore regular heartbeat and breathing tempo and to avoid overfatigue.

WARNING SIGNALS

Before going beyond a casual physical warm-up, you must learn to recognize your body's warning systems.

Any stress (physical or mental) induces a progressive reaction from one or more of the body systems. An "alarm reaction" is set off, and then fatigue, tension, or pain result.

The symptoms of stress might be shortness of breath, weakness or nonfunctioning of muscles, laziness or apathy, tension, or light trembling. If you disregard these warnings and persevere in your actions, real exhaustion may result.

When you sense an alarm signal, it is time to rest and change your exercise or rhythm in order to regain the pleasurable sensation of activity.

RELAXATION

To keep your body and mind alert and to add incentive to everything you do, you often need stimulation. But too much stimulation may create tension and fatigue. Therefore relaxation becomes a must. Any physical, mental, or emotional overexpenditure may leave you tense, irritable, exhausted, and unable to relax naturally. There are different ways to relax; the correct way can eliminate all traces of tension or fatigue.

If you sit, lie, nap, or sleep, you are relaxing passively, because you are making no physical effort. And although your circulation and other body functions slow down while your body rests, often your mental processes continue and tension may remain. Passive relaxation does not always relax you completely.

If you walk, run, jump, or exercise, you are recharging your batteries while the motor is running. By so doing you are helping to eliminate toxicity or fatigue —and you are relaxing actively. Your breathing and your circulation are increased and your mind is refreshed, relieving your nervous tension.

You can relax actively only by undertaking some form of exercise that is without the strains that produced the original fatigue, stress, or tension. Many sports or games (such as golf) do not offer enough time in motion in relation to the nervousness they induce. Only a vigorous physical activity that creates chemical changes in the body to dissipate the mind's tensions will relax you positively.

Exercising the regions of the body where tension accumulates (the neck, upper back, lower back, spine) relieves the knots in your nerves and muscles.

When active and passive relaxation fail to produce relief, some people resort to artificial methods to calm their nerves—from a simple soporific (soothing music, dimmed lights, amusing diversions) to more extreme measures such as alcohol or sleep-inducing drugs (to be used with medical approval only). These latter methods have a counteraction—a depressing weakening effect—and when used repeatedly, they produce damaging results.

PHYSIOLOGICAL CHECK-UP

THE GO-AHEAD SIGNAL

A medical check-up is essential for anyone embarking on a fitness program. In all likelihood, your body is quite ready to benefit from pleasurable exercise. But your physician is best qualified to detect any reason why you should not exercise, should there be one.

I remember the woman who arrived at my studio straight from the physician's office, bewildered. "The doctor told me I was in perfect health," she exclaimed, "but I just don't feel healthy." She sensed, as so many others have, that something was wrong but that her doctor had failed to detect it.

There is a great difference between being really healthy and simply not being unhealthy. The medical arts can help us detect and cure specific illnesses, but we can be technically free of disease and still not truly vigorous.

To a great extent body systems function unconsciously, through the sympathetic nervous system. Nevertheless, well-chosen exercises can greatly improve your respiration, circulation, digestion, and many other systems by stimulating the specific muscles involved to do their work properly. A sensible exercise program is in fact preventive medicine against breakdowns of the human machine.

Being in shape pays off in many unexpected ways. "You know the fit person on the operating table!" has been stated many times. My students have reported the startling disappearance of headaches, a decrease in colds, and the vanishing of many other aches and pains once their exercise programs are well under way.

TAKE A LOOK AT YOURSELF

The image you see reflected in your mirror is the most usual way to check personal fitness. But unless you do it properly, this can be a distressing as well as misleading way of evaluating yourself. The mirror may not show you the many other elements—besides weight loss or gain (which you read on the scale) and weight redistribution—that affect your appearance.

So many exercisers, eager for beauty, worry wrongly about their figure problems alone. They decide on a desirable weight (or series of measurements) for themselves and make this their crucial goal. As they soon learn, you cannot change your exterior unless you change the interior as well.

Pointing to himself, one friend informed me, "I want to take off 2½ inches there and 3 or so here." Another said, "I must get down to a size 9 before New Year's Eve—or else." One novice who was overconscious of her vital statistics moaned, "I can't bother with the whole fitness program. . . . All I need to do is lose 5 pounds so I'll be perfect for the beach." What she was forgetting was her need to look sleek and well proportioned as well as slender and, even more important, her need to be energetic and skillful enough to enjoy an occasional swim.

Changes in weight and proportion are most worthwhile *when they are part of a total fitness program.* You can and will make these important figure corrections for yourself as you proceed. But losing pounds is useless unless you also lose tension and fears, and thus enjoy being seen.

In other words, appearance depends on a variety of vital aspects, and you shouldn't ignore any of them in the struggle against the scales. Without excellent carriage, for example, a person with even a perfect figure will neither be noticed nor look his or her best. Being sway-backed or graceless often affects the way the world sees you far more than do excess inches.

Allure depends on more than meets the eye. It depends in fact on complete fitness. Beauty products are no substitute for glowing health; they can only enhance what is already there.

The simple aesthetic tests that follow will show you how to rate the muscle tone or firmness of your body, your complexion, posture and gait. Watch yourself in motion and analyze the appearance you project. What you see will reveal many aspects of your personal appearance that you might not have noticed before; they are vital aspects of your fitness goals.

AESTHETIC TESTS

Stand relaxed. Wear as little clothing as possible, no belt, no shoes. Take your weight and write it down._____

Take your height in inches: Standing with your back to the wall, place a telephone book vertically on your head, the spine of the book downward. Then edge the book straight against the wall and make a mark at the bottom of the book. Measure the distance from the floor to the mark._____

Because of differences in structure—differences in lengths of neck, legs, and arms as well as in type of body frame—there are variations in the relationship between height and weight. These may be as much as 15 pounds for women and 25 pounds for men.

Based on my innumerable test cards, the following charts may serve as a

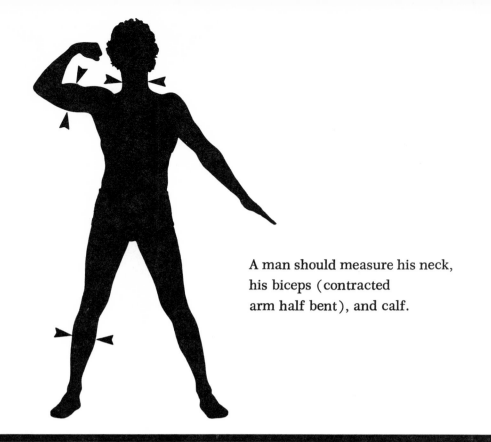

A man should measure his neck, his biceps (contracted arm half bent), and calf.

guide to appreciating and achieving an aesthetic (slim and fit) as well as healthy appearance:

HEIGHT AND WEIGHT

Women   Starting height 60 inches . . . . average weight 110 pounds
Add 3 pounds per inch. _____
(*Note that your weight may vary as much as 3 pounds in the same day.*)

Men   Starting height 62 inches . . . . average weight 125 pounds
Add 5 pounds per inch. _____
(*Note that your weight may vary as much as 5 pounds in the same day.*)

VITAL MEASUREMENTS

Women   Chest (widest circumference): _____
Waist (smallest circumference): _____
Hips (largest circumference): _____

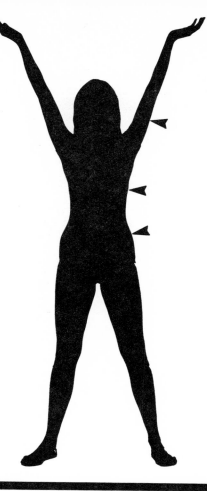

Pinch Test

Gently pinch the back of your upper arm,
the dorsal area of your ribs, and
the upper area of your hips (the areas
indicated with arrows).
If you can grasp more than an inch,
you need to firm and trim down.
But remember, women should avoid
overdeveloped muscles.
Men need muscular tissues but not
exaggerated overdevelopment.

Ideally the waist measurement should be 8 to 12 inches less than the hip and chest measurements.

Men   Neck: _____
         Biceps: _____
         Calfs: _____

Ideally the three measurements should be identical for the right proportions.

Chest (widest circumference): _____
Waist (smallest circumference): _____

The difference between the chest and waist may vary from 6 to 16 inches; the greater the difference, the better.

Posture and Gait Test

Analyze the image you project as you sit, stand, turn, walk and run.

THE SIXOMETRIC TESTS

By testing all six fitness essentials, you can determine exactly where your strength and weaknesses lie. You may be oversupple or far too stiff; you may have strength without endurance or even endurance without sufficient strength. Or you may be so close to your own top condition that a few special exercises will do the trick.

The following tests can be taken to determine your level for each of the six factors. There are some notes of caution: between your medical check-up and the time of the Sixometric tests you may have some small reasons to postpone the testing. These reasons may be minor surgical or dental operations, or minor infections like a cold, running nose, or sore throat, or indigestion, mild indisposition, a light injury preventing free movements, or an elevated temperature.

When conditions are favorable for attaining the most accurate results, perform each test in a relaxed mood and calm atmosphere, without straining

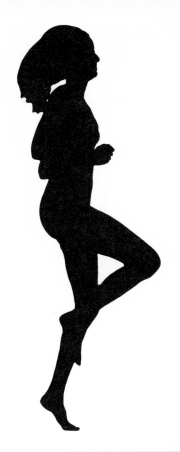

or forcing. Unless you can use each factor spontaneously, you are not performing at your best. Each test is designed to measure, in a quick and easy way, your six factors in their natural state. You will then be able to use the test results to "program yourself" to fitness. Mark the results on the score boards pages 29, 30, 36, 37, 42, 50, 51, 54, 57.

ENDURANCE

When taking a long walk, climbing two flights of stairs, performing errands, or doing a simple chore like washing the windows brings on any sign of fatigue, you are revealing a lack of endurance.

Endurance is the factor that helps your energy last over a long period of time, and you call upon it constantly. Long-distance runners and swimmers, and all durable performers are able to perfect their endurance by undergoing specialized training. By improving your lung capacity and breathing patterns as well as strengthening your heart muscles, you can train yourself to resist fatigue and make anything you do easier, from driving great distances to dancing through the night.

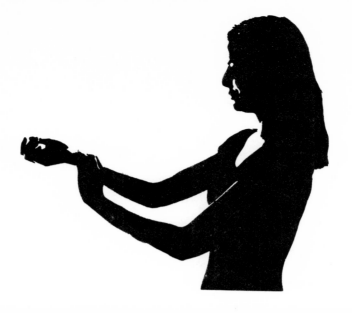

Tests for Endurance

Our heart and lungs are the most important organs of endurance. Try the following tests:

1. PULSE RATE

At rest in a reclining position. Press the fingertips of one hand gently to the inner wrist of the other, and count the number of pulsations of the artery in one minute. A man's pulse rate should be approximately 70 to 75 beats a minute or less. A woman's, 73 to 78.

If you are really at rest with no worry or hurry and your pulse rate is 10 to 15 beats higher than the norms given, it could simply be the effect of tobacco or coffee, or some other reason. It is wise to recheck your physical condition with your doctor.

2. HEART RESPONSE

Test your heart response to vigorous movement. The best time for the test is in the morning before breakfast and before smoking—if you do!

Sit for 5 minutes, take your pulse, and mark it down. Then perform 10 knee bends in 20 seconds. Sit down, take your pulse every minute, and mark it down, until your pulse rate is restored. Your pulse rate should be restored in 3 minutes or less.

You may also, especially if you feel fitter, perform the following exercises to keep a record of your improvement.

Skip a rope or run for a minute. Record your pulse rate. Every time you take the test keep the same skipping rhythm or running pace for the identical period of time.

Or perform a more vigorous exercise.

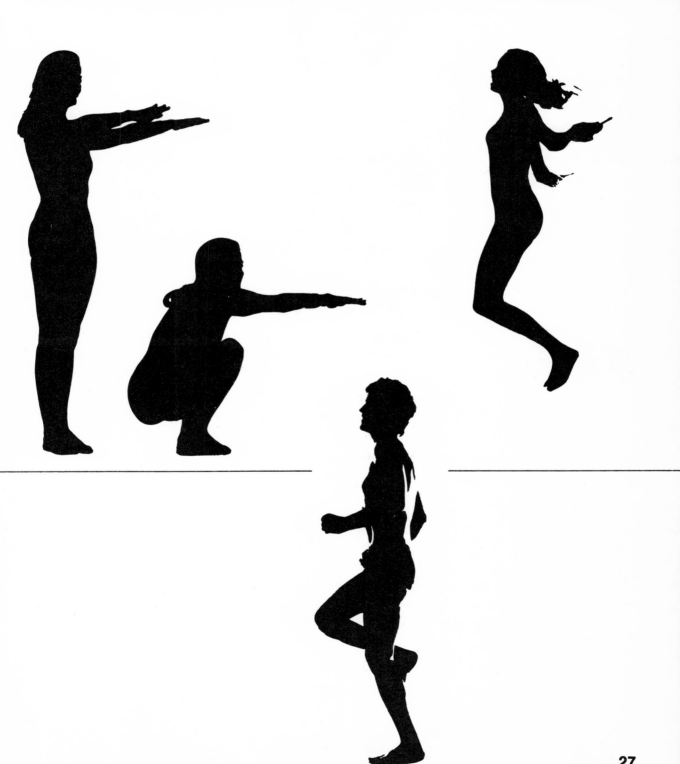

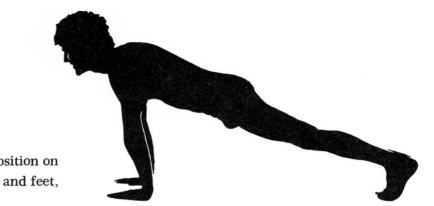

From a support position on
your hands and feet,

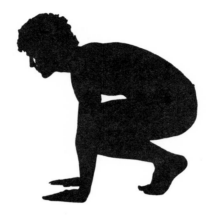

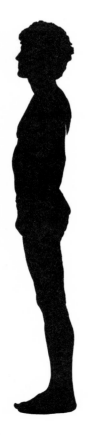

swiftly lifting your hips,
jump to a crouch position and
immediately stand up.
Reversing the movement, return
to the support position.
Repeat the exercise 10 times
in 20 seconds. Take your pulse,
note how long it takes
to restore the regular heartbeat
or pulse rate.

The quicker the return to normal, the better. If it takes more than 5 minutes, your endurance is poor.

It is interesting to notice that after a reasonable period of proper training your pulse rate recovery time shortens, sometimes to a minute or less.

These simple tests emphasize the importance of gradual programming. Vigorous or strenuous exercises must be avoided until you are ready for them.

3. LUNG CAPACITY

Proper breathing is vital to your endurance. Besides learning the correct way to breathe, you should know your lung capacity, that is, the volume of air you inhale and exhale with each breath.

The simplest test is to take a deep breath, hold it in, and measure your chest with a tape measure. Then exhale as much as possible, hold, and measure your chest again.

The difference between the two measurements should be at least 3½ inches for men and 2½ inches for women. The greater the difference, the better.

To rate yourself tops in endurance you should be able to swim, run, play an active sport, or dance for several hours without any symptoms of fatigue.

Unless you can pass the above tests with ease and a natural smile, your resistance to fatigue is probably inadequate and you need to improve your endurance.

SCORE BOARD

Test One: Pulse rate

Women	72 beats per minutes or less	}	good
Men	70 or less		
Women	From 72 to 78	}	fair
Men	70 to 75		
Women	Over 78	}	insufficient
Men	Over 75		

Test Two: Heart response

Men and Women	Less than 2 minutes	good
	From 2 to 3 minutes	fair
	Over 3	insufficient

Test Three: Lung capacity

Women   Over 3 inches   good
               From 2 to 3 inches   fair
               Below 2   insufficient
   Men   Add 1 inch to all figures

YOUR ENDURANCE SCORE

Test One	Test Two	Test Three

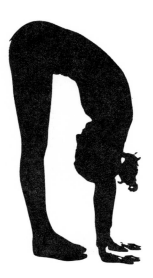

SUPPLENESS

Getting into a car, picking flowers, bowling, playing with young children, or simply swinging a tennis racket requires a certain flexibility, because all these activities involve some bending, arching, or twisting. Therefore, you need suppleness in the joints of your body.

You can increase your flexibility through practice. Unless a trained athlete exercises specifically for limberness, he may become unmanageably stiff ("muscle bound") while a weak, slim, or even plump person who is physically untrained can be so supple as to be almost collapsible.

Many things may affect a person's degree of flexibility, among them physical characteristics, state of tension or relaxation, and even the surrounding temperature.

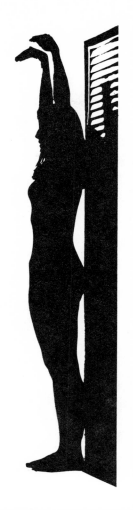

Stand with your back
against a wall,
shoulders, back, hips,
and heels touching
the wall.
Raise your arms
forward and up, wrists bent,
and try to touch the wall
with your wrists.

Tests for Suppleness

1. SHOULDERS

The smaller the distance between your wrists and the wall, the more supple your shoulders are. If the distance is more than 10 inches, your shoulders are pretty stiff, and you must avoid exercises involving suspension from a bar or other apparatus until you have improved your flexibility.

2. FORWARD SUPPLENESS OF SPINE

Sit on the floor, legs together and straight, toes pointed. Bend forward, without forcing, and try to touch your toes with your finger tips.

The distance between your finger tips and toes reflects your forward suppleness. Measure the distance for future reference.

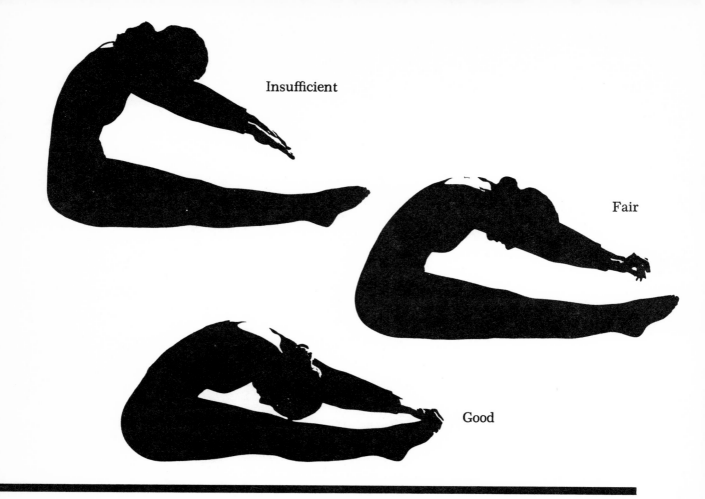

Insufficient

Fair

Good

3. BACKWARD SUPPLENESS OF SPINE (*Women*)

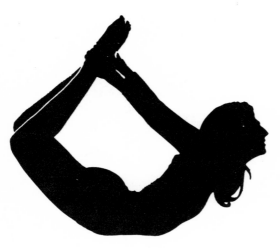

Lie on your abdomen,
bend your knees,
and try to grasp your ankles.
Then, without forcing,
arch your spine.

NOTE: A man's muscular development usually interferes with the backward flexibility of his spine, but most women, if they are fit, should be able to do this test. If you can get your shoulders and knees 10 to 12 inches off the floor, your backward suppleness is adequate.

4. LATERAL FLEXIBILITY

Perform the exercise as if you were sliding against an imaginary wall.

Standing with legs far apart, arms up, hands together

bend your body to the right, left arm stretched in a prolongation of your body, right arm tucked behind your back.

Repeat the same exercise, bending to the left, changing arms.

5. TWISTING

Sit on the floor, legs apart,
toes pointed, hands
clasped behind your head.

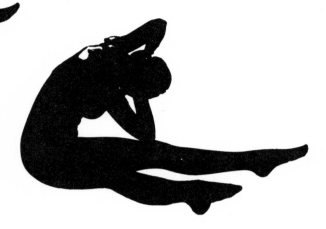

Gently twist your trunk
to the left, and try to touch your
left knee with your right elbow.
Then twist to the right
and try to touch your right knee
with your left elbow.

If you can touch each knee with the appropriate elbow, you are flexible enough. If you cannot, note the distance between knee and elbow.

---

6. PIVOTING

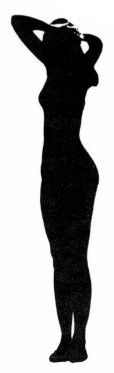

Imagine you are
the center of a clock face.
Stand, feet together,
facing straight ahead, hands
clasped behind your head.
Slowly twist your
spine to the right and, looking
over your right shoulder,
try to see four o'clock.

Twist to the left
and try to see eight o'clock.

7. HIPS (Primarily for *Women*)

Stand and raise your right arm forward, the hand slightly above the level of your head, the other arm back for balance. Swing your right leg forward and try to touch your right hand without bending your knees or lowering your hand. Then try the test with your left arm and leg.

Note the distance between your toes (pointed) and your hands.

If you cannot raise your leg above the horizontal, your hips are not supple enough.

If your leg is 45 degrees above the horizontal, your hips are supple enough.

If you touch your hand with ease, you have excellent suppleness in your hips.

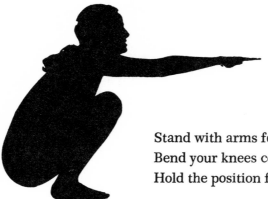

Stand with arms forward, feet flat on floor.
Bend your knees completely, crouching down.
Hold the position for a few seconds.

8. HIPS, KNEES, AND ANKLES

If you cannot perform the above tests with ease and freedom, your suppleness is inadequate. Be sure to warm up sufficiently before attempting any difficult exercise.

If some of your joints are not supple enough, you will not be able to do certain exercises fully or freely, and they will be less effective.

Remember: suppleness has no age limit, and only inactivity induces a stiffening of joints and limitation of movement.

SCORE BOARD

Test One: Shoulders

Touching the wall	good
Less than 6 inches	fair
Over 6 inches	insufficient

Test Two: Spine (forward)

Overlapping toes	good
Less than 10 inches	fair
Over 10 inches	insufficient

Test Three: Spine (backward) (*Women*)

Free arch, no pull	good
Ankle grasp, knees and shoulders 5 inches off the floor	fair
Difficulty in grasping ankles	insufficient

Test Four: Lateral Flexibility

Over 80 degrees	good
45 to 80 degrees	fair
Less than 45 degrees	insufficient

Test Five: Twisting

Touching	good
Up to 6 inches	fair
Over 6 inches	insufficient

Test Six: Pivoting

180 degrees, both sides (6 o'clock)	good
120 degrees (4 o'clock and 8 o'clock)	fair
Less then 120 degrees	insufficient

Test Seven: Hips (Primarily for *Women*)

Approaching your hand	good
A foot away	fair
Over a foot away	insufficient

Test Eight: Hips, Knees, and Ankles

Complete flection, easy position	good
Complete bend holding on to a chair	fair
Inability to reach position	insufficient

YOUR SUPPLENESS SCORE

Test One	Test Two	Test Three	Test Four
_____	_____	_____	_____

Test Five	Test Six	Test Seven	Test Eight
_____	_____	_____	_____

BALANCE

To walk through a moving train or perform tasks from the top of a ladder, you must have perfect balance or suffer the consequences. Whether you are

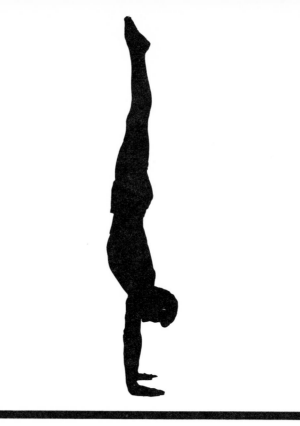

moving or at rest, you need your sense of orientation and equilibrium to keep your balance.

As soon as you begin to lose your balance, your sense of equilibrium (controlled by the semicircular canals and the cocklea, and coordinated by the cerebellum and the spinal cord) detects the cause and corrects it. The more perfect is your equilibrium, the more gracefully and easily you are able to move.

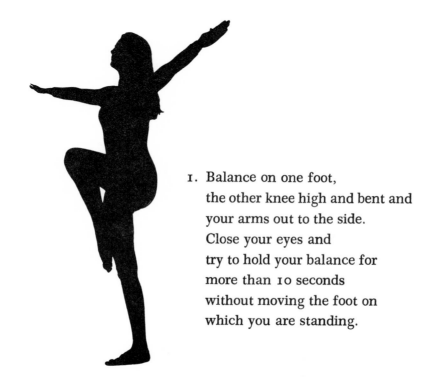

1. Balance on one foot,
   the other knee high and bent and
   your arms out to the side.
   Close your eyes and
   try to hold your balance for
   more than 10 seconds
   without moving the foot on
   which you are standing.

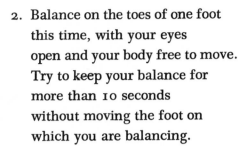

2. Balance on the toes of one foot
   this time, with your eyes
   open and your body free to move.
   Try to keep your balance for
   more than 10 seconds
   without moving the foot on
   which you are balancing.

3. Stand on one foot and bend
   forward with arms stretched out
   to the side and one leg
   held back and high. Try to hold
   the position for 10 seconds.

4. Balance on your hips with
   your arms and legs raised as high
   as possible, contracting your
   abdominal muscles. Maintain perfect
   balance for 10 seconds.

Tests for Orientation

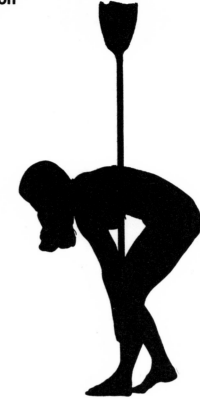

5. Press one end of a broomstick
   to the floor, bend over it,
   and, grasping the stick
   close to the bottom,
   press it to the floor.
   Using the stick as a center pivot,
   walk around it 6 times.
   Then release the stick and walk in
   a perfectly straight line.

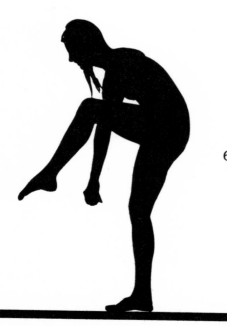

6. Walk on a beam or
   4-inch-wide line with a
   yardstick held in your hands.
   Pass one foot over the
   stick and bring it back without
   losing your balance.

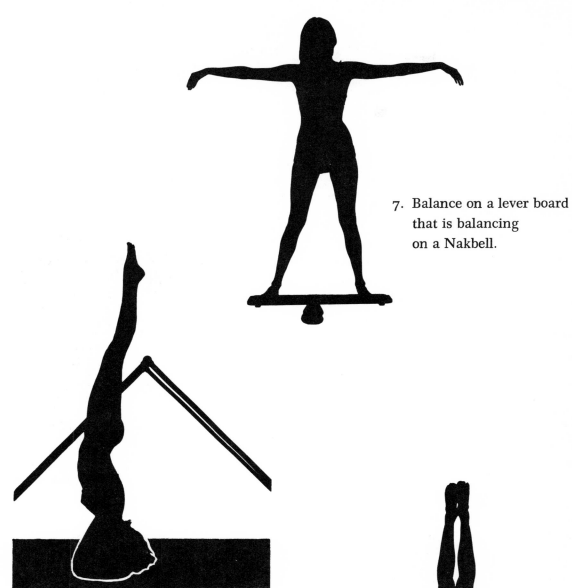

7. Balance on a lever board
   that is balancing
   on a Nakbell.

8. Balance upside down
   (only for experts).
   Supporting yourself.
   Headstand.

9. By suspension
   (inverted hanging)
   from a Nakbar.

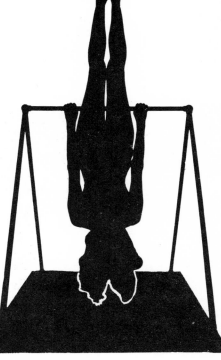

SCORE BOARD

Tests One to Four:

10 seconds or over	good
Between 5 and 9 seconds	fair
Less than 5 seconds	insufficient

Tests Five and Six:

Easy straight walk	good
Effort to maintain straight walk	fair
Wobbling walk	insufficient

Test Seven:

Easy balance for over 30 seconds	good
Balance from 10 to 30 seconds	fair
Less than 10 seconds	insufficient

Tests Eight and Nine:

10 seconds or over	good
From 5 to 9 seconds	fair
Less than 5 seconds	insufficient

YOUR EQUILIBRIUM SCORE

Test One	Test Two	Test Three	Test Four	Test Five
_____	_____	_____	_____	_____

Test Six	Test Seven	Test Eight	Test Nine
_____	_____	_____	_____

STRENGTH

When you move furniture, take a big dog walking in the park, or even open a stubborn jar, you need strength. A person who appears to be muscular may still be quite weak. In fact a slender, tense individual may well be stronger than someone larger and more threatening-looking.

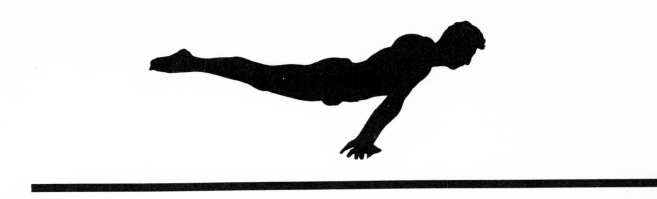

Your strength depends on the precise quality of your muscles, and it may be hereditary or acquired through training. It is a factor that must not be over-emphasized in any physical program; a man can become "muscle bound" and not be able to use his strength. And highly developed muscles make a woman unattractive.

But a woman should still be able to lift packages or a child, or open a jar without undue strain. A man should be able to lift his own weight with ease, climb a rope using only his hands, and carry heavy luggage or another person.

Strength wisely developed as part of a total fitness program will serve you well. You must practice constantly to maintain it. When you work on your strength factor, your flesh stays firm, your muscles toned, and your figure and posture are at their best.

Tests for Strength

1. ARM EXTENSORS (*Men*)

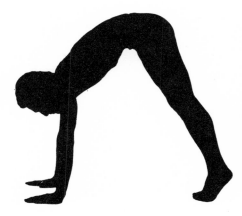

Stand with your back
to the wall and your heels
touching the wall.
Bend over and place your hands
on the floor at a distance
away from the wall equal roughly
to half your height.

Keeping your legs straight,
do 6 complete push-ups.

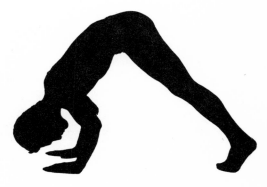

2. ARM FLEXORS (*Men*)

Grasp the frame of the door or the branch of a tree, and, with your feet off the ground, try to chin yourself 6 times without jerking or kicking. Or try the Nakbar:

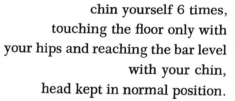

Sitting on the floor and holding the bar, knees bent with feet off the floor,

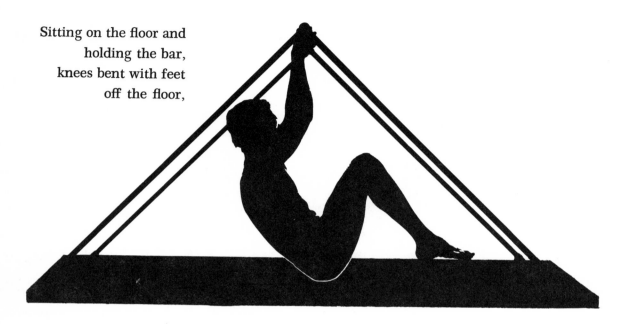

chin yourself 6 times, touching the floor only with your hips and reaching the bar level with your chin, head kept in normal position.

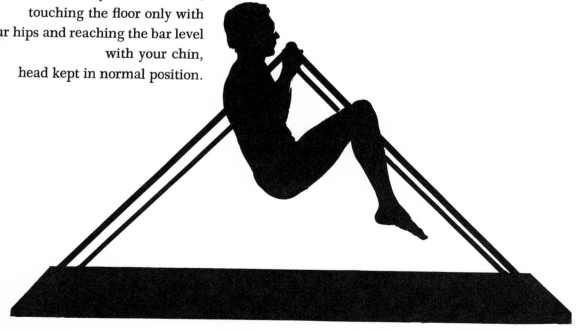

3. FINGER FLEXORS

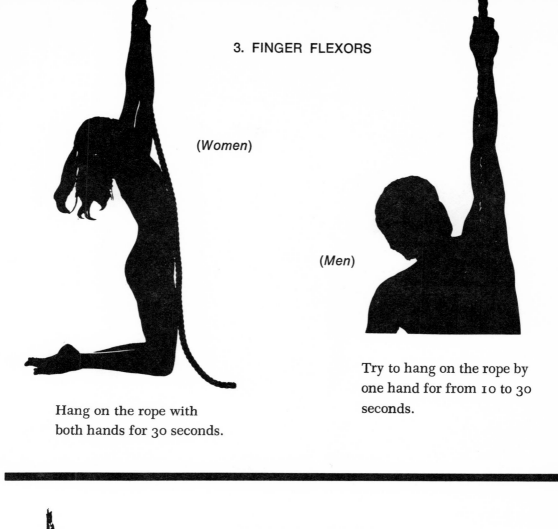

(Women)

(Men)

Try to hang on the rope by one hand for from 10 to 30 seconds.

Hang on the rope with both hands for 30 seconds.

4. ABDOMINAL STRENGTH

A. Lie on your back, arms up, legs straight.

Slowly try to sit up; do this 6 times.

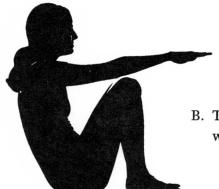

B. Try the same exercise starting
   with your knees bent.

C. Balance on your hips
   keeping your back, legs, and arms
   off the floor and maintain
   that position for 30 seconds.

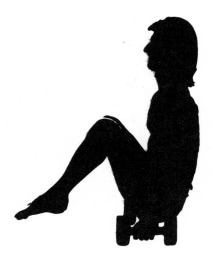

D. (*Men*) Using two Nakbells
   or two telephone books, support the
   weight of your body on your
   hands and arms only.
   Try first with your knees bent
   and hold 6 seconds.
   (A difficult exercise; do not
   strain yourself.)

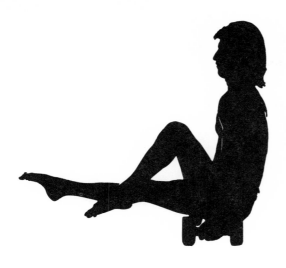

E. (*Men*) Then try the same test
with one leg straight
and one bent.

F. (*Men*) And finally try it with
both legs straight.

---

5. CHEST AND ABDOMEN (*Men*)

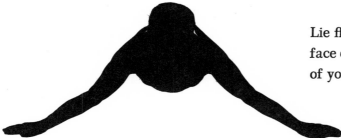

Lie flat on the floor,
face down, arms stretched in front
of you and wide apart.

Press down and try to lift your body
off the floor so that only
your hands and feet are touching it.
Hold the position for 10 seconds.
(Another difficult exercise;
do not strain.)

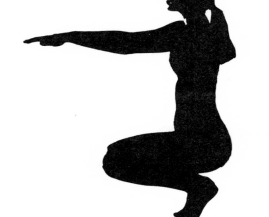

6. LEGS

Stand on your toes
against a wall or door,
with your arms in front of you.
Keeping your back straight,
slowly bend your knees and squat.
Then slowly rise, sliding
against the wall or door.

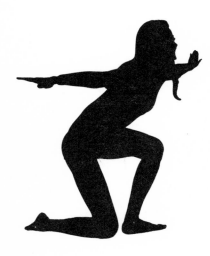

7. ONE LEG

(*Women*) Kneel on one leg,
keeping the foot of
the kneeling leg off the floor.
Using the power of
the other leg, try to get up
without allowing the lifted foot
to touch the floor.

(*Men*) Arms in front,
holding weights or Nakbells
as a counterbalance,
with the left leg in front
of you, slowly try
to squat and then stand up,
bending and straightening
the right leg.
Try to do the same exercise
bending the left leg.

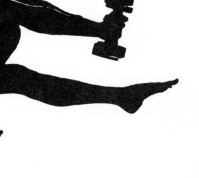

SCORE BOARD

Test One: Arm Extensors (*Men*)

6 push-ups and over	good
Less than 6 push-ups	fair
No push-ups or longer distance from wall	insufficient

Test Two: Arm Flexors (*Men*)

Over 6 times	good
3 to 5 times	fair
Less than 3 times	insufficient

Test Three: Finger Flexors

Women	30 seconds or over	good
	From 10 to 29 seconds	fair
	Less than 10 seconds	insufficient
Men	Same scoring	

Test Four: Abdominal Strength

Men and *Women*	Doing C easily	good
	Doing G easily	fair
	Doing only A or less	insufficient
Men	Doing D easily	good
	Doing E easily	fair
	Doing only F or less	insufficient

Test Five: Chest and Abdomen (*Men*)

Reaching and holding position with arms straight	good
With arms half-bent	fair
With hands close to shoulders	insufficient

Test Six: Legs

10 times	good
5 to 9 times	fair
Less than 5 times	insufficient

Test Seven: One Leg

Women	Doing it with ease	good
	Doing it with help	fair
	Not being able to do it	insufficient
Men	6 times with ease	good
	From 1 to 3 times	fair
	1 or none	insufficient

YOUR STRENGTH SCORE

Test One   Test Two   Test Three   Test Four

_____   _____   _____   _____

Test Five   Test Six   Test Seven

_____   _____   _____

SPEED

Whether it's a work deadline, a close tennis match, or a bus to be caught, you need speed to perform rapid body movements. This factor helps you do anything quickly or under pressure to the best of your ability. The faster the muscles obey the nerve impulses they receive, the faster you can physically respond.

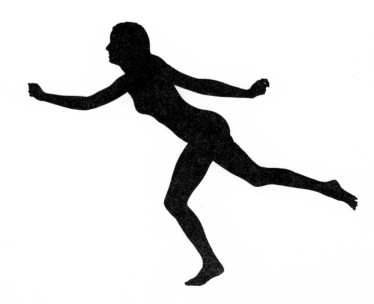

Speed may refer to an isolated action of a part of your body, such as the legs or the forearms, or to the combined action of areas of the body, as in racing or swimming.

If you feel you are in good shape, test yourself in a 100-meter dash and compare your time to the 10 seconds that is the men's record or the 11 that is the women's.

If you can get into a fast revolving door easily, catch a fast ball, grasp a tow rope on the ski slope, you have adequate speed.

Besides being a lifesaver, should you have to dodge a reckless driver or avoid a falling object, speed is useful in countless daily tasks and in all active sports. However, speed is one factor that requires careful control or you will "overstrain your own brakes" or swing too quickly and miss your aim. Your speed needs adjusting in any sport as well as each time you rush during a pressured day.

There are two types of speed: *initial speed,* which helps you activate a movement, initiate a fast action; and *maximum speed,* which is the highest pace or fastest action that your body may produce.

Strong, well-conditioned muscles will help you move faster (unless they have been overtrained or overdeveloped, in which case they slow down the action).

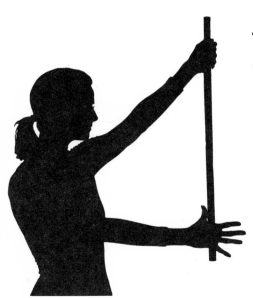

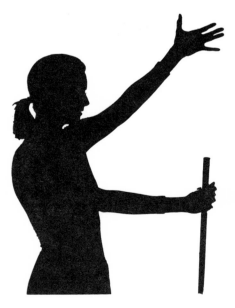

Tests for Speed

1. INITIAL SPEED

Hold the top of a yardstick with one hand, leaving the other hand open and close to the bottom of the stick.

Release the grip of the upper hand, and as the stick drops, try to catch it with the lower hand.

The point at which you catch the stick indicates your initial speed.

If you catch it at less than 20 inches, your initial speed is pretty good.

To be accurate, this test should be done with someone else holding the yardstick and dropping it and with your own arm on a table with the hand overhanging the edge.

2. MAXIMUM SPEED

Pin a sheet of paper on the wall or door about 10 inches above your head.

Stand sideways, one foot from the wall, legs approximately 25 to 30 inches apart.

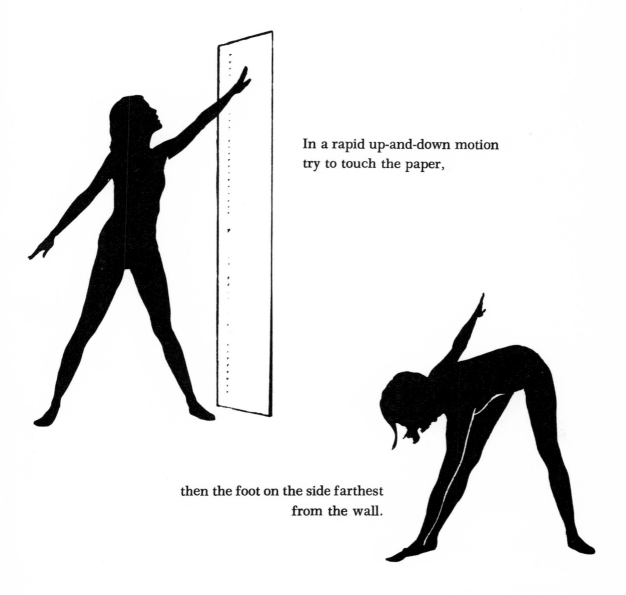

In a rapid up-and-down motion try to touch the paper,

then the foot on the side farthest from the wall.

Repeat the complete movement 10 times in less than 10 seconds and you are pretty fast!

3. FOR EXPERTS ONLY

Try to run a 60-meter dash.

SCORE BOARD

Test One: Initial Speed

Catching it immediately	good
Catching it halfway	fair
Barely catching it	insufficient

Test Two: Maximum Speed

10 times in less than 6 seconds	good
10 times in 6 to 10 seconds	fair
10 times in over 10 seconds	insufficient

Test Three: For Experts Only

In less than 8 seconds	good
In 8 to 10 seconds	fair
In over 10 seconds	insufficient

YOUR SPEED SCORE

Test One	Test Two	Test Three
_____	_____	_____

COORDINATION

The final reward for the perfection of the preceding factors is coordination.

We see exciting examples of human coordination on the stage, in the sports arena, and wherever we ourselves execute simple or complex movements.

By means of coordination, we function harmoniously and precisely. Without it, endurance, suppleness, equilibrium, strength, and speed are useless—just as the most perfectly built car is useless without a driver.

When you are well coordinated, specific skills such as skiing or mowing the lawn seem far less taxing than before.

Because a child hasn't perfected this factor, he moves and performs awkwardly, with a great deal of wasted effort.

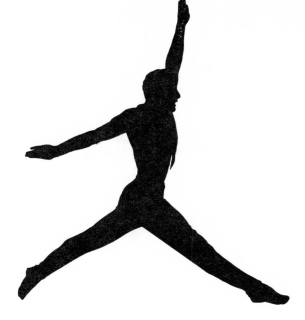

Through evolution, man has lost the natural sense of coordination that every member of the animal kindgom still possesses. A bird, after all, can learn to fly in a matter of hours. Only man is obliged to practice to acquire muscular skills, and he may lose the skill if he doesn't stay in practice.

You must learn to coordinate all your movements so that you use the minimum effort for a given task. Everyone can improve his coordination. With dedication an awkward youngster with weak arms and no stamina can become a champion.

Tests for Coordination

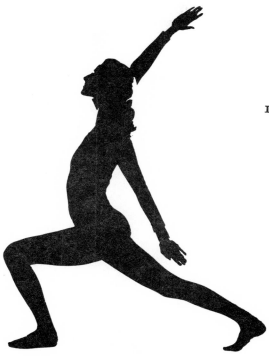

1. Stand with your feet together, then lunge forward with one leg while raising the arm on the opposite side. Return to a standing position and immediately lunge with the other leg, while raising the opposite arm. Repeat 6 times.

2. Bend your body to the side.
Balancing yourself, stand
with your right leg
and left arm horizontal and
your right arm raised.
Slowly, without losing balance,
reverse the positions of
your arms and legs.
Do the exercise 6 times
without mistakes and without
losing your balance.

3. Stand facing forward,
then lunge to the right side, bounce,
raise the right leg high,
and return to standing position.
Repeat on the other side,
and continue, alternating right and
left sides. Do this 6 times,
lifting your leg higher each time.

4. Can you easily learn a new dance, play a game of tennis, swim, skate, or ride a bike?

Do you drive without tension?

Can you hold a tray of tall drinks in stable balance? Walk with ease in a moving bus?

Do you feel comfortable in an upside-down position?

SCORE BOARD

Executing all the tests and excelling in Test Four	good
Executing all the tests but not excelling in Test Four	fair
Having difficulty with any of the tests	insufficient

YOUR COORDINATION SCORE

Good	Fair	Insufficient
_____	_____	_____

PSYCHOLOGICAL EVALUATION

MENTAL FITNESS: AN INTERIOR EXAMINATION

We live in a world that demands not only endurance but also mental keenness, not only speed but also resistance to overbearing tensions, and not only a radiant image but also clear thinking for innumerable complex decisions. Your physical make-up alone reveals only part of the story. Psyches vary as greatly as physiques. Physical weaknesses often develop as a result of mental attitudes and emotions. Our minds control and affect every action we perform. I have seen how correct exercise promotes positive psychological changes in everyone who undertakes the Sixometric program, from the bored housewife to the overtense corporation president.

Physical and mental fitness nourish and support one another. For this reason, your exercise program can be geared to correct many psychological or emotional problems. An elderly but active man recently remarked, "My morning exercises are the only thing that really puts my thoughts and my body together." Psychologists and psychiatrists often specifically recommend exercises to their patients, giving this kind of therapy their highest approval. "A patient can sometimes work out problems in your studio that might take him years on a couch," one doctor told me recently.

Take a few moments to analyze yourself. Are you too demanding of yourself, or perhaps too lax? Do you have trouble releasing pent-up emotions, or coping with tensions? Is it hard for you to feel "collected" and secure within your own body? Many people lack the ambition or the confidence to undertake new projects or to follow tasks through to the end. Are you rigid in your ways, or too pliant? Do you rush needlessly, or are you afraid of spontaneous movements? In countless cases I have seen the right exercises correct many psychological limitations, sometimes greatly to the student's surprise.

THE FACTORS OF SUCCESS

If you proceed rationally, it is not only possible to improve every one of the six factors—it is inevitable. A seventy-year-old who exercises will have far better mental and physical endurance than an inactive young man, and this rule applies to many facets of our daily life. Each one of us has anatomical and physiological limitations, of course, but we are all still capable of achieving far more than we do. Judging from thousands of novice students, anyone will tend to expect far too little of himself unless he is proven wrong. And engineered exercises are designed to prove that you have underestimated your six factors, and yourself.

Make a point-by-point analysis of the factors your currently favorite sport or exercise improves. Does it really help you to withstand daily tensions and traffic, as well as to enjoy a full and active life with complete mental and physical coordination and endurance? Whatever the activity, it should help you gain endurance (improved with prolonged activity) and keen coordination (improved through the performance of a variety of movements). It should also engage some physical strength (more for men) as well as make use of your equilibrium, flexibility, and speed.

In my estimation, only the most carefully designed exercises will improve each of the above factors pleasurably, in the minimum amount of time. Programmed engineered exercises are designed to make you fit for all seasons, games, and life goals.

A well-regulated program such as this accomplishes far more than even a large number of strenuous but haphazardly chosen exercises. Each exercise can be performed as a natural movement, and each leads to a further, more demanding physical accomplishment. The correct dosage also prevents you from overexercising, a common error in many gymnasiums and studios. Those who overdo may end up less fit than they were when they began and thus accelerate the aging process.

Some slogans worth remembering are:

While young you may be physically old!
Middle age may come at any time!
Physical old age may be by-passed!

And a great slogan of the American Health Foundation is: *Die young as late as possible!*

No one sport can assure you the all-around benefits of a personal exercise program, which can become as stimulating, pleasant, and rewarding as any athletic activity. As a student of mine once stated, "With such personal exercises, you are always on the winning team."

Sixometry is the system I suggest to attain these goals, but my real faith is in you—the exerciser. Can you spare 6 minutes a day—less than an hour a week —for enjoyable self-improvement? Optimally, you should practice engineered exercises at least twice a week, and judging from the experiences of my students, you will soon want to. These few minutes can change your life.

A woman whose throat is firm and young will feel youthful and self-assured. The man with bolstered stamina will do a better day's work with less effort, and he will enjoy his leisure with renewed vigor. Tennis scores will improve, and so will marriages. Those of us who experience greater pleasure are able to give this same pleasure to others. And this is perhaps the most important joy that comes from feeling fit.

Sixometry carries over into every aspect of life. When our bodies are totally adjusted, we feel more integrated and generally competent. Learning to control ourselves in any position within the 360-degree range helps us overcome fears and begin to enjoy physical activity and the positive forces of life more fully. The more we enjoy movement, the more beautifully we move.

When you exercise Sixometrically, you avoid exhaustion and the unsatisfying or boring forms of physical activity. While machines need only careful engineering to maintain their fitness, man needs *enjoyable* engineering to maintain his.

BEFORE YOU BEGIN

As a first and foremost rule, if you have been inactive for a long time (or if you are a beginner at exercising), proceed as if you were a convalescent. This might sound overcautious, but unmoderated action often leads to physical setbacks rather than progress. You cannot be too conservative where your body is concerned.

Select surroundings that suit you. Well aerated rooms with high ceilings prove best. The area should be clean, pleasantly lit, and at a comfortable temperature.

The best time to exercise depends on your personal preference and daily schedule, but try to choose a time that you can keep *regularly*. Regular activity is far more beneficial than sporadic work; a 5-hour session once a month is not enough and much too harsh.

A set schedule is the easiest way to be faithful to your fitness program. You should never be rushed, or your concentration and relaxation will suffer.

Never exercise directly after meals.

Wear clothing that permits you free, comfortable movement and allows your skin to breathe as well.

Pleasant but not overpowering music or a pace-setting device like a metronome is the easiest guide to follow for tempo. Remember that any interruption can affect the continuity of your exercise session. Do try to avoid midexercise telephone calls.

Exhale through your mouth with your lips half closed; inhale through your nose, nostrils remaining wide open. Windows can be opened for additional fresh air.

Choose exercises that involve all parts of the body, separately as well as together.

Use muscles both individually and in groups, in all types of contractions.

Move in all directions and positions, using every one of the six factors.

Remember that an overdose or the wrong kind of effort can lead to negative results. You may overtax your motor system when all you wanted was an overhaul, or develop muscular bulges where they are not needed. It is possible to tighten up rather than loosen up, or stimulate when you prefer to relax.

Proceed with care and gentleness. Your body's natural functions and mechanics are highly complex and are easily affected by any change in routine. You may not realize how intricate your glands, joints, circulatory system, and muscle fibers are until you start your fitness program.

Begin by performing small amounts of exercise; increase this number gradually but never to the point of fatigue. Moderation is the key to successful exercise as well as fitness.

In addition to rhythm, each movement demands a certain effort in order to be useful to the body. Exercising with slightly increased intensity will permit you to progress to a higher degree of fitness.

Finally, to insure that each session brings you the most benefit, you must plan the exercises in the right order for you, allowing for brief rest periods within the session. You should always, for example, begin with the setting-up exercises and follow with posture exercises, no matter what the rest of your program is.

Just as it takes anyone a certain amount of time to learn a new talent (such as how to walk or drive a car), *exercising becomes easier as you practice.* Once you have initiated a program for fitness, it will eventually become a natural part of your life, as well as a beneficial and enjoyable part of your day. Gradually, your proficiency will improve along with your health. But because I'm convinced you will notice the satisfying effects of your program at once, healthful exercising will soon become as vital to you as meals and rest.

Each new skill involves specific factors and will take concentration and patience to achieve. Some skills will come more naturally than others. It is wiser to perfect your physical abilities gradually within a total fitness program than to try to display premature technical feats without a basically fit condition to sustain them. Don't forget that your most worthwhile goal is not a perfect headstand but to live each moment of life with ease, health, and pleasure.

EXERCISE AESTHETICS

One of the most valuable secrets of successful exercise is to *look attractive at all times.* Without fail, a pleasant appearance in practice clothes improves what you see in the mirror, your attitude about what you are doing, and your morale. Unfortunately, looking just right in leotards or practice shorts is often the last thing one thinks of while exercising, and it should be the first.

I remember the time I proved this theory. It was in my studio in Paris; I greeted a number of students ready for class and noticed how unsightly their long gym bloomers made them appear. Quite impetuously, I grabbed a pair of scissors and trimmed off the entire line of bloomer legs to expose attractive legs and enliven the room. The week after, the number of participants doubled.

Today, practice clothes are usually more becoming. Make sure you look your absolute best before you begin to move.

Motion can—and should be an attractive habit. Physical action promotes one's best health and physical functioning, of course; but we often forget that the quality of our movements directly affects almost every aspect of our lives, from social success to the daily level of energy and the enjoyment of activity of all kinds.

It is my conviction therefore that there is only one way to exercise—beautifully. Each motion in an exercise can easily be learned and performed in the most effortless, graceful, and efficient way possible. Furthermore you will soon be able to execute daily tasks, sports, and spontaneous movements with the same ease and beauty, as well as increased inner satisfaction.

To master beautiful exercising, you should study the written instructions and the illustration of each exercise carefully, and follow the rhythm indicated. In most instances the head should follow the direction of the spine and not be thrust forward; the upper back should be straight but at the same time partially relaxed to give freedom of action; your muscles should be contracted just enough to perform the exercise.

Keep your toes pointed in the direction of the movement, hands and arms graceful, and your expression, if not joyful, at least pleasant. By all means avoid a tense expression or exaggerated breathing and puffing.

Once your exercise program has been planned, with the dosage and procedure based on your Sixometric test scores and your body type, plus your innate masculinity or femininity, you will understand as well as feel the value of your own pleasure in motion.

PLANNING YOUR PERSONAL DOSAGE

How much exercise you will enjoy doing will depend on which category you belong in at this time. Are you a beginning, intermediate, or advanced exerciser? This may be determined by your calendar age, your physical age, and above all, the length of time you have not engaged in vigorous physical activity.

Calendar age is important but physical age has priority. You can be old at twenty-five and young at sixty-five—it depends on your health and fitness. Nevertheless if you have not exercised recently or participated in any active sport or work, you are a beginner—even if you are an inactive sportsman or sportswoman.

If you are an active person and have passed the Sixometric tests—above all, the endurance tests—without failure, you should be capable of performing the beginner's program with ease. Consider yourself an intermediate.

If you are a sportsman or sportswoman and have been exercising regularly, and if you passed all the Sixometric tests with ease and can indulge in an active sport or dance and run or climb with no sign of shortness of breath and excessive heartbeat, consider yourself advanced.

For each category there is a daily exercise series planned for your convenience. Each series includes the essential movements you need to perform to insure yourself maintenance and improvement of fitness—even if you have an irregular life schedule.

Your Personal Procedure

Each exercise that you are going to perform can be done six different ways, depending on which factor you wish to stress. Refer to your scores on the Sixometric tests and regulate your program according to your specific needs. If you have insufficient or only fair

ENDURANCE: Exercise with moderation, paying special attention to your breathing. Increase gradually, avoiding speed until your endurance improves.

SUPPLENESS: Perform each exercise completely—increasing the range of motion, gently forcing the stretch, and relaxing completely in between.

EQUILIBRIUM: Supplement your exercise by performing it balancing on one foot or on your toes, and with your eyes closed.

STRENGTH: In each exercise emphasize each contraction—beginning with resistive effect (eccentric contraction), then holding effect (static contraction), then overcoming effect (concentric contraction).

SPEED: Perform your exercise as swiftly as you can, accelerating to reach the maximum speed.

COORDINATION: Vary your performance by exercising in all the previous styles, in different order and combinations.

PROGRAMMED FITNESS

In following your personal dosage and personal procedure, you may find that certain weaknesses will be overcome sooner than others as your program goes along, but this is natural. Once every factor is brought up to its most desirable level, you will see your level of efficiency rising. As you improve, your fitness standards will rise as well.

Now is the time to harmonize your exercising with your body type and avoid a program that in the long run might prove unsuitable and unrewarding.

Guidelines for Body Types

Appraising the characteristics of your predominant type (page 5), select the most appropriate manner in which to do your long-range exercising.

The ectomorph type should eat a well-balanced diet in a relaxed, pleasant atmosphere; in addition, he should be sure to chew his food slowly and well, which will allow his body sufficient time for digestion.

The ectomorph should exercise his underdeveloped body areas thoroughly, using a slow rhythm and making sure to complete all muscular contractions and relaxations. By breathing deeply and moving without tension, he will gradually increase his strength and form new muscle fibers. An ectomorph's exercising must always be accompanied by complete and frequent rest periods. He needs pampering: soothing music and pleasant surroundings. Above all, he should avoid extreme temperatures and disturbances during his exercise sessions. This kind of exercise will improve his metabolism, permitting his body to absorb more nutritive substance and gain more benefit from the food he consumes.

The endomorph type tends to turn almost everything he absorbs into fatty tissue, making it hard for him to lose extra weight. Scientists report that to lose weight by diet alone may lead to unfitness. Lack of exercise is almost as bad for your weight as overeating and may be worse for your health and appearance.

Localized exercising helps "burn up" the areas that need reduction. But correct exercise involves strategy: While legs may be too heavy, they should be worked carefully so that muscles do not develop. If hips need reducing, isolated hip movement should be accentuated. Strategically engineered exercise is the best way for endomorphs to eliminate fatty substances, firm their muscles, and reduce general body volume.

Keep in mind that any radical change in nourishment or activity can weaken your system. Drastic diets or physical overexertion might remove the protective fatty tissues that cover, warm, and help to support the body. Food quantity can be decreased, but a balanced diet must be maintained to avoid malnutrition.

An endomorph should exercise slowly at first to build up his endurance; then he must gradually increase the rhythm, quantity, and intensity of his exercises. Eventually he should increase the physical activity in his daily life as well.

The mesomorph type (mostly male) can decrease the unnecessary energy he expends for given tasks in order to improve his physical efficiency. With proper breathing and a slight moderation of food intake, a mesomorph can counterbalance his excessive activity and become more relaxed. He should exercise for coordination, working at a moderate pace and emphasizing skill and free expression. In this way his positive characteristics will be used to advantage.

To accentuate her femininity, a female mesomorph should strive to decrease her muscular development. Firm muscular tissues are difficult to reduce; she should exercise in a relaxed manner, accentuating all graceful movements. Specific posture exercises and softly rhythmical motions can be useful. Above all she should avoid energetic gestures and static or "holding" muscular contractions.

To sum up: We must keep ourselves from appearing either weak to the point of fragility or solid to the point of immobility. The aesthetics of physiology must prevail with the emphasis on suppleness in women and strength in men.

ENGINEERED EXERCISES (GYMNAKS)

What you are going to begin may be the most important project you have ever devoted yourself to.

It is worthwhile starting correctly, guided by the golden rules of Sixometry to prevent discouraging effects and to insure efficiency.

Your body will welcome the exercises as a mental and physical delight as well as preventive medicine or therapy.

If any one of the described exercises seems difficult at first, perform only a part of it, such as a slight knee bend instead of a full knee bend, progressing gradually to the full exercise.

At the start repeat each exercise twice, increasing by one every two or three days, until you reach 6 of each.

Follow the rhythm indicated in the exercise.

Interspace your exercise session with deep breathing pauses of a few seconds.

Try to exercise every day; if not, every second day is still good.

To maintain fitness a minimum of once a week is necessary.

If you exercise less than once every ten days, fitness begins to fade away.

DOSAGE FOR THE BEGINNER

1. Setting-up Exercises   Series A, 1 to 12
2. Minimum Daily Sixometrics   Series G, 1 to 6
3. Winter Exercises   Series J
4. Relaxation
5. Deep Breathing

(The winter exercises may be done in bed or on the floor. They are mild and good for circulation.)

Gradation-Progression—Daily Quota

First two days   Each exercise 2 times
Third day   Each exercise 3 times
Fifth day   Each exercise 4 times
Seventh day   Each exercise 5 times
Ninth day   Each exercise 6 times

(If the progression of every two days feels a little strenuous, protract the increase to every week. For someone who has not exercised for a long time, it may take from six weeks to six months to get into the groove of fitness.)

DOSAGE FOR THE INTERMEDIATE

1. Setting-up Exercises   Series A, 1 to 12
2. Posture   Series B, 1 to 3
3. Waistline and Back   Series C, 1 and 2
4. Balance and Relaxation   Series D, 1 and 2
5. Strength (*Women*)   Series E, 1 and 2
   Strength (*Men*)   Series E, 1 and 2
6. Stretch (*Women*)   Series F, 1 to 3
   Stretch (*Men*)   Series F, 2 and 3
7. Medium Daily Sixometrics   Series H, 1 to 6

8. Exercises for the Appropriate Season:
   Winter   Series J
   Spring   Series K, 1 to 3
   Summer   Series L, 1 to 3
   Fall   Series M
9. Relaxation
10. Deep Breathing

Each of the stipulated setting-up exercises should be done 6 times. For all other exercises, follow the gradation-progression scale in the beginner's section.

DOSAGE FOR THE ADVANCED

1. The Entire Fitness Session   Series A to F
2. Maximum Daily Sixometrics   Series I
3. Exercises for the Appropriate Season   Series J to M

Add Minimum Daily and Medium Daily Sixometrics

(Naturally exercises selected for men should be avoided by women to eliminate the chance of developing a masculine characteristic. As for men—all exercises may be attempted, taking care not to overdo the suppleness exercises.)

FITNESS SESSION

SETTING-UP EXERCISES

For the best distribution of blood throughout the entire body, begin the session by using those muscles that are the farthest from each other—starting from the extremities of the body and progressing to the central or waistline region.

Proceed without unnecessary tension but nevertheless totally contract and then relax each set of muscles.

Breathe normally as you exercise, exhaling through your mouth, inhaling through your nose.

Perform the movements rhythmically to the tempo of 50 beats a minute (larghetto).

1. Hands

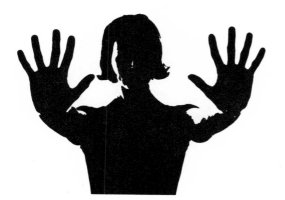 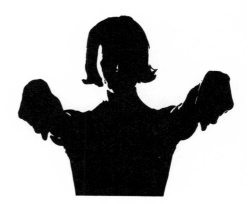

Arms in front of you
at shoulder level, bend your
hands up so the palms are
facing forward and spread your
fingers wide.

Bend your hands down
and curl your fingers tight.

---

2. Feet

Place your hands
on your hips and rise
on your toes.

Rock back to your heels.   And lift your toes.

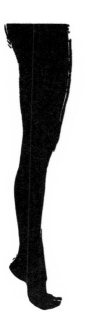

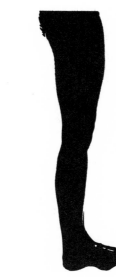

3. Neck

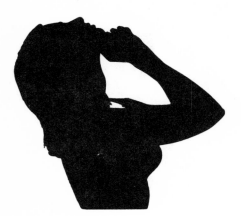

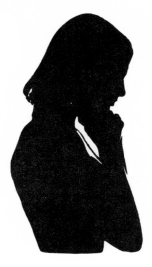

Cover one fist with
the other hand and, pressing
against your chin, move your head
up and back. Inhale.

Still pressing your chin
against your fists, move your head
forward and down. Exhale.
Your neck should resist the pressure
of your fists each way.

4. Legs

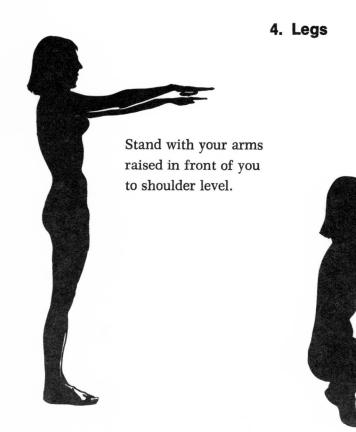

Stand with your arms
raised in front of you
to shoulder level.

Keeping your heels
on the floor, bend forward
slightly and squat.
Exhale as you squat,
inhale as you rise.

5. Chest

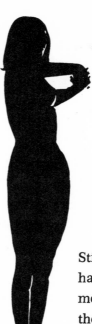

With your arms raised
to shoulder level,
your elbows bent, and the
heel of one hand pressing
against the other,
move your arms to the right.
Keep facing forward.

Still pressing one
hand against the other,
move your arms to
the left.

6. Hips

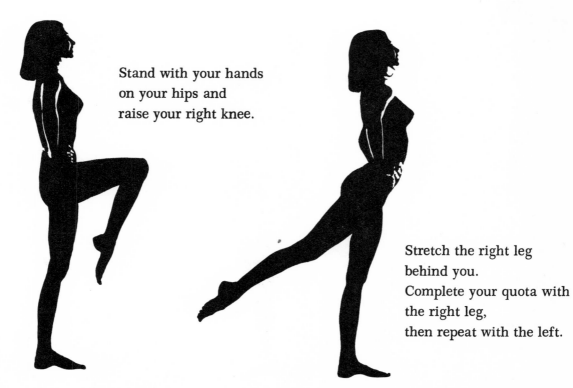

Stand with your hands
on your hips and
raise your right knee.

Stretch the right leg
behind you.
Complete your quota with
the right leg,
then repeat with the left.

7. Shoulders

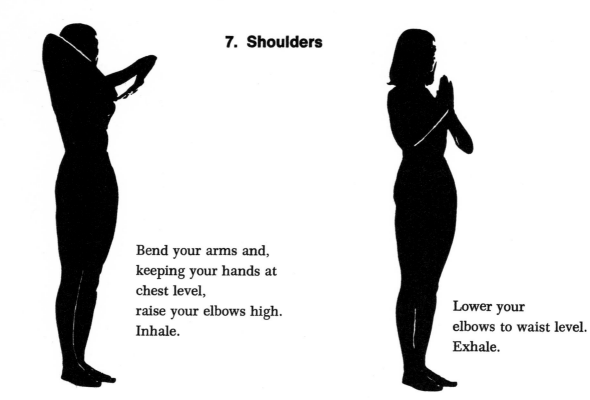

Bend your arms and,
keeping your hands at
chest level,
raise your elbows high.
Inhale.

Lower your
elbows to waist level.
Exhale.

8. Abdomen and Chest

Clasp your hands behind
your head.

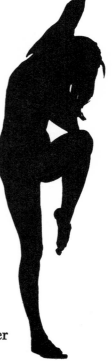

Raise your right knee
and lower your left elbow,
trying to join them.
Exhale as you bend, inhale
as you straighten up.

Then raise your
left knee and lower
the right elbow.

9. Back and Hips

Stand with your legs
apart and your hands clasped
behind your head.

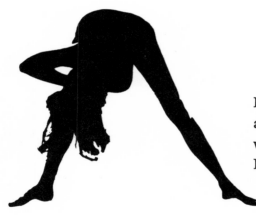

Bend forward, twisting,
and try to touch your right knee
with your left elbow.
Exhale as you bend down.

As you straighten up, inhale.
Then repeat, trying to
touch your left knee with
your right elbow.

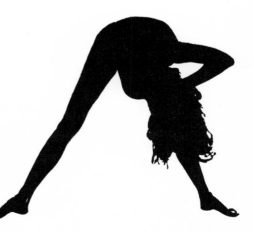

10. Waist

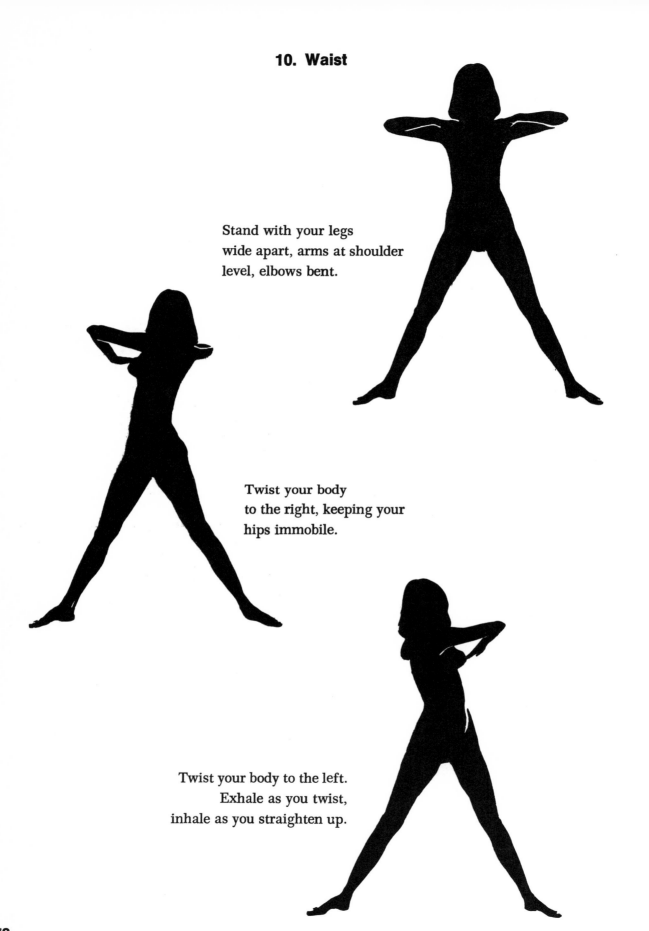

Stand with your legs
wide apart, arms at shoulder
level, elbows bent.

Twist your body
to the right, keeping your
hips immobile.

Twist your body to the left.
Exhale as you twist,
inhale as you straighten up.

11. Stretch and Relax

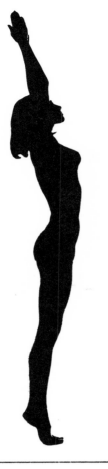

Raise your arms sideways
until they meet above your head,
and at the same time slowly
rise on your toes and stretch high.
Inhale 6 beats.

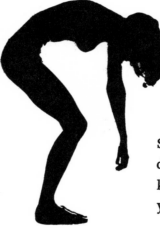

Slowly drop your arms
down sideways, and bend your
knees and back. Exhale as
you go down, 6 beats.

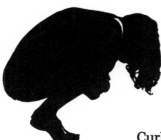

Curl your body into a crouch,
hugging your knees.
Repeat the entire sequence twice.

12. Coordination and Breathing

Crossing your arms, exhale.

Spreading your arms
describe a wide circle with
them while raising
one knee high. Inhale,

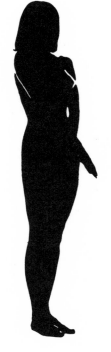

cross your arms again,
then continue circling your arms.
Lower the knee and repeat
the sequence with the other leg.
Repeat 6 times.

POSTURE EXERCISES

As soon as the setting-up series is completed, with muscles warmed up and joints loosened up, perform the posture exercises.

They will set the body in its best posture and carriage for the entire session.

In performing these exercises emphasize extension, gently forcing corrective positions, and follow a slow tempo of double 50, with 2 beats for each movement.

1. Standing with your legs wide apart, raise and spread your arms. Inhale.

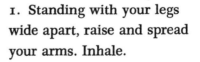

Then slowly bend forward and cross your arms. Exhale.

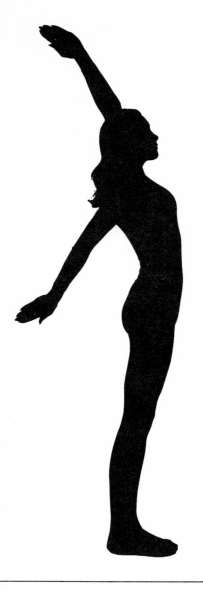

2. Standing straight,
   raise your right arm up and
   back and bring your
   left arm down and back.

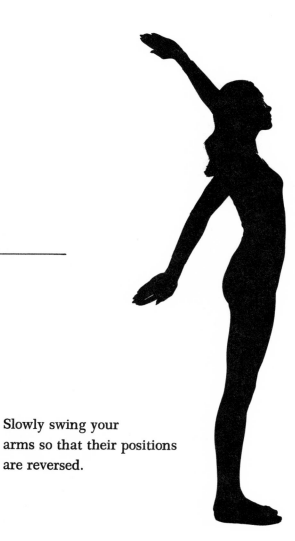

Slowly swing your
arms so that their positions
are reversed.

Slowly bend forward
at the waist, keeping both your
arms as high as possible.

3. Stand with one arm
held straight in front, and
the other straight back.

Then slowly bring both
arms together in front of you.

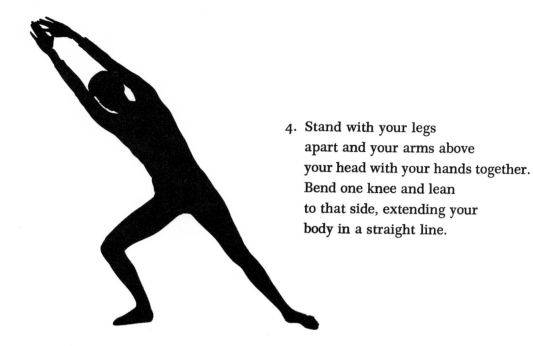

4. Stand with your legs
apart and your arms above
your head with your hands together.
Bend one knee and lean
to that side, extending your
body in a straight line.

Repeat the exercise
bending the other knee and leaning
to the other side.

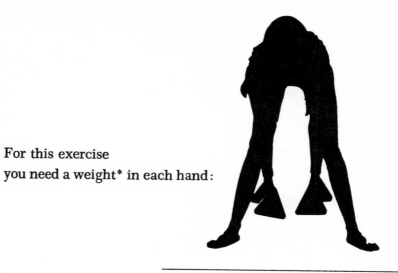

5. For this exercise
   you need a weight* in each hand:

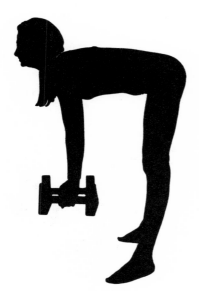

one of 2 pounds for women and
one of 6 to 10 pounds
for men. Body bent forward,
keeping your head up
and back straight, your arms
hanging down,

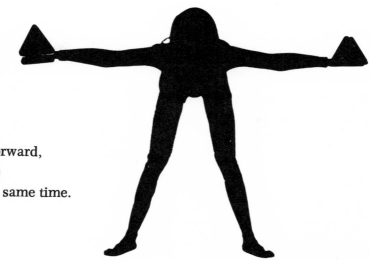

raise your arms to
the side, slightly forward,
so that you can see
both weights at the same time.

* See page 182.

6. Sit on the floor,
   with your arms behind you,
   leaning on weights* or
   telephone books.

Slowly raise your hips and
arch your back.

Hold this position 6 seconds,
then bend one knee.
Hold for 3 seconds and then
sit down slowly.
Repeat with the other leg.

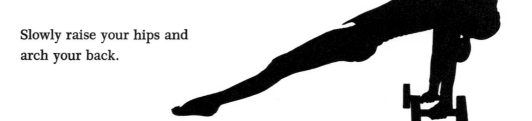

* See page 182.

86

WAISTLINE AND BACK EXERCISES

Next come the important central muscles of the waistline and back. To firm your abdominal girdle, to slim down your waistline while limbering your spine, hips, and shoulders, perform these exercises with complete contractions and synchronized breathing.

Exhale when the chest is compressed, inhale when it is expanded.

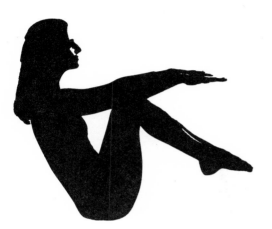

1. Balance on your hips with your knees bent, feet off the floor, and arms forward.

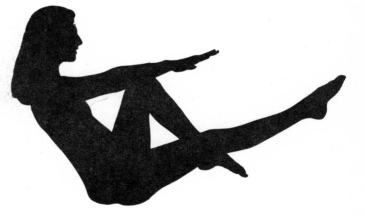

Slowly extend one leg and then bend it.

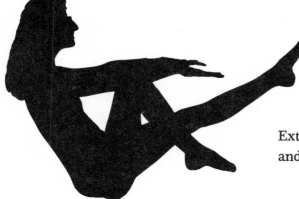

Extend the other leg, bend it, and continue, alternating legs.

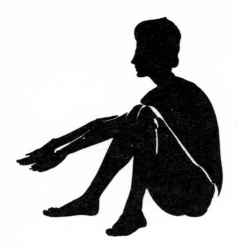
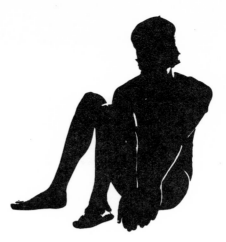

2. Sit on the floor
with your arms forward,
knees bent, and feet apart.
Turn the upper part of
your body and move
your arms to the right.

Gently lean back,
turn your body, and move
your arms to the left.

3. Sit on the floor with
your right knee bent and your arms
at shoulder level, elbows bent.
Twist your body and try to
touch your right knee with
your left elbow. Complete your
quota on the same side.

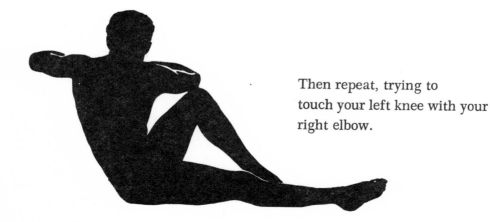

Then repeat, trying to
touch your left knee with your
right elbow.

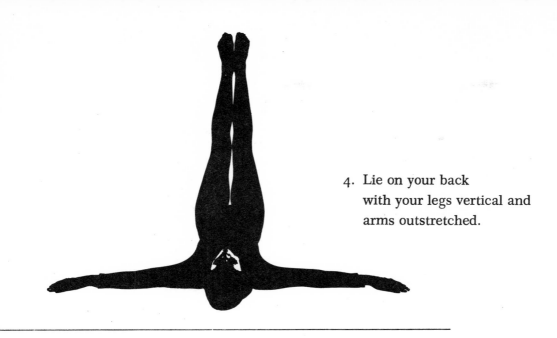

4. Lie on your back
   with your legs vertical and
   arms outstretched.

Slowly lower your legs
to the left.
Then raise them.

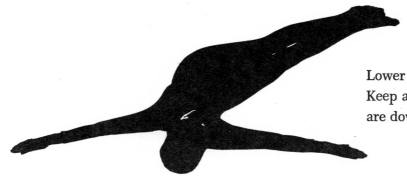

Lower your legs to the right.
Keep alternating—exhaling when legs
are down, inhaling when up.

5. Lie face down on the floor
   with your arms stretched in front
   of you. Slowly raise your
   right arm and left leg
   as high as possible.

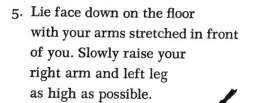

Repeat with the left arm
and right leg. Inhale when the leg
and arm are up, exhale
when they are down.

6. Lying face down on the
   floor, arms forward, raise
   your arms and legs simultaneously.
   Complete your quota—
   inhaling while your limbs
   are up, exhaling
   while they are down.

BALANCE AND RELAXATION

To relax and change the pace, perform an easy feat of balance or coordination; it will give you a chance to recuperate.

Learn a new skill—a dart game, cup and ball, juggling, or the following exercises.

1. Sitting on the floor, on a carpet or mat* (to avoid bruising your vertebrae), bend forward until your hands touch your toes. Exhale deeply.

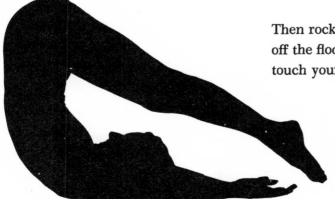

Then rock back, hips off the floor, until your toes touch your hands.

* See page 182.

2. Lie on your back, arms bent,
   palms flat on the floor.
   Breathe normally.

Raise your legs and hips.

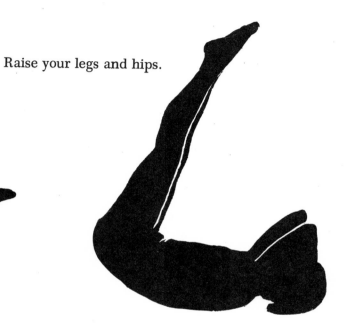

Balance on your upper back,
neck, and hands,
keeping your legs straight.

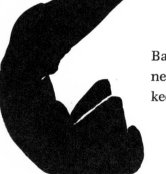

Touch the floor behind you
with your left leg.
Then with your right leg.

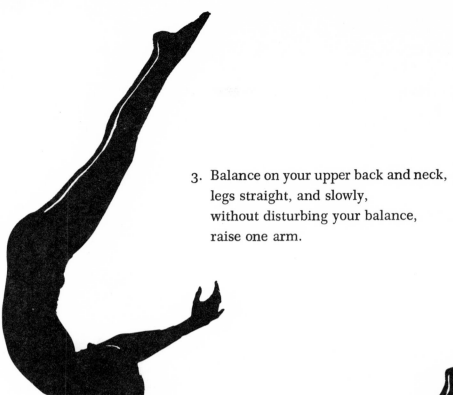

3. Balance on your upper back and neck,
   legs straight, and slowly,
   without disturbing your balance,
   raise one arm.

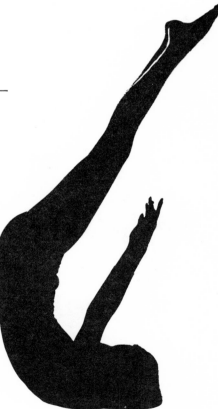

Raise both arms.
Breathe deeply for 6 seconds
and come down.

STRENGTH EXERCISES FOR WOMEN

Women can keep trim and add grace to their movements by exercising their hips, thighs and legs. These exercises improve flexibility of the hip joints and supply necessary activity to a rather inactive region.

Follow a tempo of 50 beats a minute (breathing regularly).

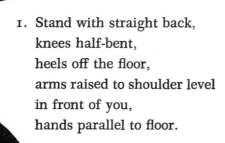

1. Stand with straight back,
knees half-bent,
heels off the floor,
arms raised to shoulder level
in front of you,
hands parallel to floor.

Straighten your legs,
putting your heels on the floor,
and raise your right leg,
bending your ankle so that your
foot is parallel to your body
and the toes are up.
At the same time bend your
wrists so that your palms
are facing forward.

Return to a half-squat
position, then straighten up,
heels on floor, and
raise your right leg again,
this time with toes pointed and
hands bent down. Repeat
the exercise with the left leg.

2. Stand with arms outstretched
   on either side at shoulder level.
   Raise your right leg
   to the side, toes pointed.

Lower your right leg
and with the same motion
raise your left leg
to the side, toes pointed. Keep
alternating legs, each
time lifting them higher and
higher without forcing.

3. Kneel on the floor and
   bend forward, supporting your
   body with both hands.
   Straighten your right leg
   to the side and lift it, as you
   balance yourself by
   raising your left arm on
   the other side.

Keeping both right leg and
left arm straight,
raise and lower the leg,
counterbalancing the movement
with your left arm.

Repeat the exercise
with your left leg and right arm.

4. Sit on the floor, arms and
   legs straight in front of you,
   and then roll back,
   raising your legs over your head
   until they almost touch
   the floor behind you. Exhale
   as you swing back.

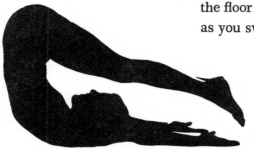

Gently swing your arms and
legs forward again and,
as you do so, bend your right
knee and put your right
foot on the floor.

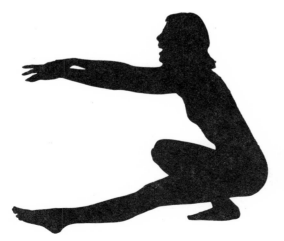

Keeping your momentum,
press with your right foot and,
slightly, with your left
heel, and try to lift
your hips off the floor.
Inhale as you swing forward.
Repeat the exercise,
alternating with the left leg.

STRENGTH EXERCISES FOR MEN

Men can add power to their arms, shoulders, neck, back and legs with strength exercises that will make their daily tasks easier, improve their appearance, and help correct postural defects.

1. Support your body on your arms
   with your feet on a chair.

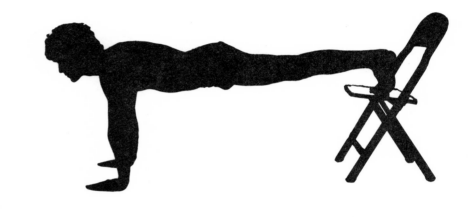

Do slow push-ups,
then fast push-ups.
Synchronize the rate of
your breathing with the rhythm
of your push-ups.

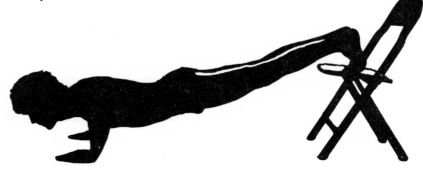

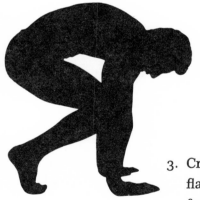

2. Stand with your right leg forward, your arms in front of you holding two weights of Nakbells.

Keeping your right leg forward, bend your left knee, counterbalancing with your weights. Straighten up and repeat with your right leg, keeping your left leg forward. Progress gradually.

3. Crouch with your hands flat on the floor, feet on the floor, supported on the toes.

Carrying your weight on your hands and arms, slowly try to raise your hips and legs, balancing on your hands.

Be sure to have a Nakmat* or pillow under your head, and, if the exercise is too difficult, try it with your feet apart, supporting your weight on your elbows.

* See page 182.

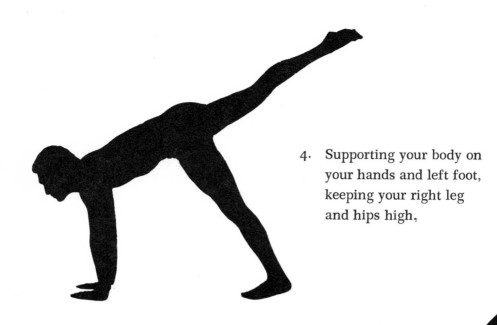

4. Supporting your body on
your hands and left foot,
keeping your right leg
and hips high,

bending your arms,
slowly move your shoulders in a
circular pattern,
first back and down,

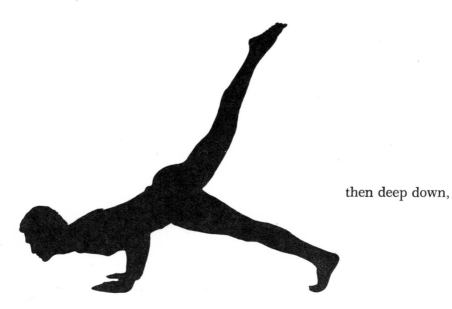

then deep down,

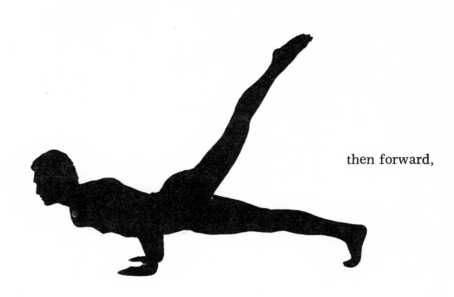

then forward,

and finally up.
Full circle one way,
then reverse—forward,
down, deep down,
backward-up, then up.
Repeat same with the left leg up.
Perform slowly—6 seconds each circle.
Breathe deeply and slowly.

STRETCH EXERCISES

To wind up the first part of the session, some stretching exercises will relieve the pressure of gravity, loosen the spine, and adjust the vertebrae.

A suspension bar in a doorway (or over the door) or a Nakbar will enable you to do certain healthful exercises from a suspended position.

The following stretch exercises do not, however, require special equipment.

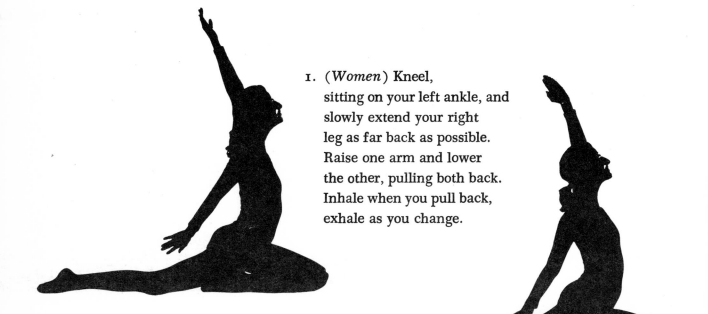

1. (*Women*) Kneel,
   sitting on your left ankle, and
   slowly extend your right
   leg as far back as possible.
   Raise one arm and lower
   the other, pulling both back.
   Inhale when you pull back,
   exhale as you change.

Reverse the arms.
Then perform the same exercise
sitting on the right ankle
and extending the left leg.

2. (*Men* and *Women*) Lie prone
   with your left arm forward,
   and raise and bend your left leg
   until you can grasp
   the ankle with your right hand.

Still holding this position,
lift your right leg and
left arm as high as possible.
Then repeat the exercise
with opposite arm and leg.
Inhale as you stretch up,
exhale when down.

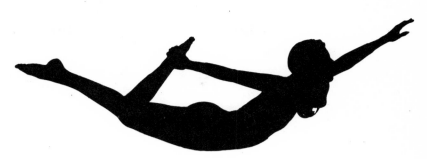

3. (*Men* and *Women*) Stand with your
legs as far apart as
possible and, arms up, grasp
your left wrist with
your right hand. Inhale.
Pull up and back, and bend your
body to the right side.
Exhale.

Straighten, inhale,
release your wrist, bend forward,
and touch the floor
with both hands, palms down.
Exhale.

Repeat on the left side,
grasping your right wrist with
the left hand.

SIXOMETRICS

MINIMUM DAILY SIXOMETRICS

To keep up with the challenges of the day and to stay symmetrically fit, perform at least one exercise for each physical factor.

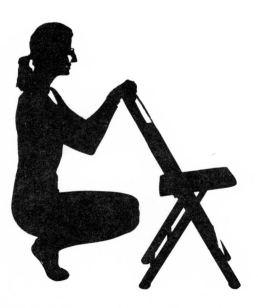

1. Endurance

Holding on to the back of a chair or a door knob, squat and straighten up. Exhale as you go down, inhale as you come up. Keep a slightly accelerated tempo, 100 beats a minute (allegretto).

2. Suppleness

Sitting on a chair
leaning against the back,
raise your arms and reach as far
back as possible.
Inhale as you raise your arms,
exhale as you bring them down.
Take 3 seconds to reach, and
3 seconds to relax.

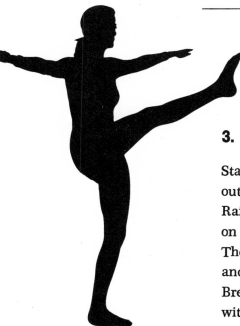

3. Equilibrium

Stand with your arms
outstretched to the side.
Raise one leg and try to balance
on the other for 10 seconds.
Then raise the other leg
and balance.
Breathe normally, try this also
with the eyes closed.

4. Strength

Lie on the floor and,
swinging your arms forward,
try to sit up halfway.
Exhale as you sit up,
inhale as you lie down.
Keep a tempo of 50 beats a minute.

5. Speed

Stand with legs apart, body bent forward
and arms stretched out at the side.
Rapidly twisting your body, try to touch the floor
first with one hand, then with the other.
Accelerate progressively to 184 beats a minute
(prestissimo) or even faster.

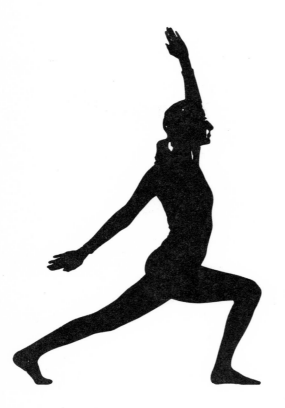

6. Coordination

From a standing position,
lunge forward with your right leg,
at the same time raising
your left arm and stretching
your right arm down and back.
Inhale as you lunge,
exhale as you return to
standing position. Repeat with
your left leg and right arm.

MEDIUM DAILY SIXOMETRICS

1. Endurance

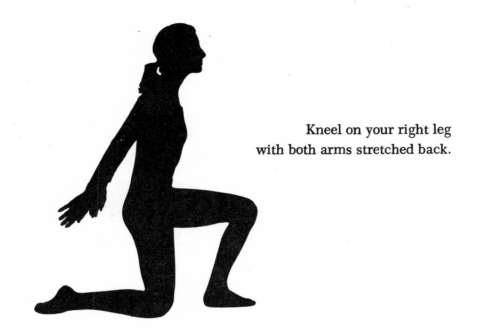

Kneel on your right leg
with both arms stretched back.

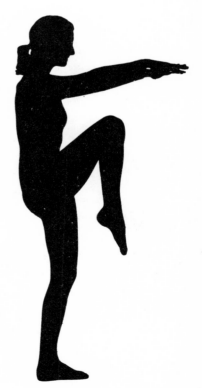

Swing your arms forward, stand,
and raise your right knee.
Then return to the kneeling position.
Repeat, kneeling on your left leg.
Inhale as you rise,
exhale as you kneel. Try to keep
an active tempo from
moderato to presto or from 80
to 144 beats a minute.

2. Suppleness

Stand with your legs together,
heels on the floor,
and then bend forward and
try to touch the floor with the
flat of your hands.
Exhale as you bend down.

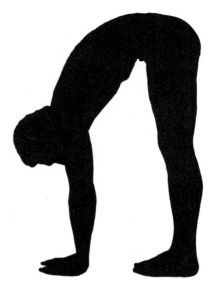

Then lunge forward on your
left leg, arching your spine and
raising your arms up
and back. Inhale as you rise.
Repeat, this time
lunging on your right leg.
Take 6 seconds for
the complete exercise.

3. Equilibrium

Stand on your right leg
with arms outstretched to the side
and lean to the right,
using your outstretched left leg
and horizontal right
arm to maintain your balance.
Hold the position for 10 seconds.

Repeat the exercise balancing
on your left leg.
Try it with your eyes closed.

4. Strength

Lie on your back
with arms and thighs up,
knees bent.

Without changing
the position of your thighs,
try to sit up and
lie down. Exhale as you rise,
inhale as you go back.
Use a slow tempo of 30 beats a minute.

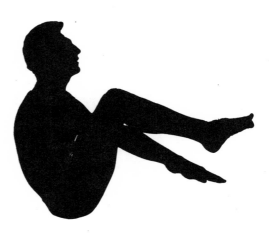

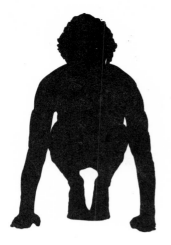

5. Speed

Crouch with your hands
flat on the floor.

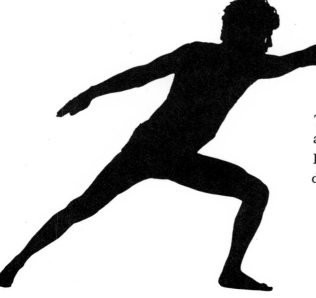

Swiftly lunge to the right,
reaching with your arm as in
a lunge in fencing.

Then return to the crouch position
and lunge to the left.
Lunge deep—extend completely and
do it as fast as you can.

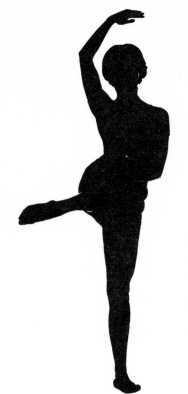

6. Coordination

Stand on your left leg,
with your right knee raised high,
your foot turned to the side,
your right arm bent
over your head, your left arm
behind your back.

Extend your right leg
to the side and up, and at
the same time, reverse the position
of your arms—the left arm
bent over your head,
the right behind your back.
Repeat, standing on your right leg
and extending your left,
starting with your left arm
over your head and
your right behind your back.

Perform at various speeds.

MAXIMUM DAILY SIXOMETRICS

1. Endurance

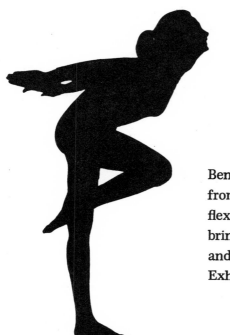

Bend slightly forward
from a standing position and
flex your right knee,
bringing your arms back
and your chin up.
Exhale.

Then extend your right leg back
and swing your arms
forward and up. Inhale.
Use an accelerated tempo of 116
beats a minute (allegro).
Complete your quota with
the right leg, then do
the same exercise, flexing
your left knee.

2. Suppleness

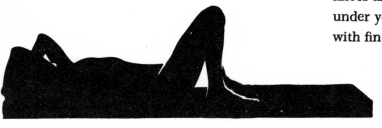

Lie on your back
(on a nonslippery surface),
knees and arms bent, palms flat
under your shoulders
with fingers in, feet apart.

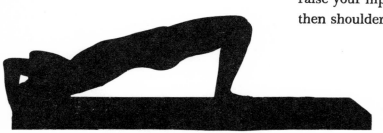

Pressing evenly with your hands and feet,
and moving your knees forward,
raise your hips,
then shoulders, off the floor.

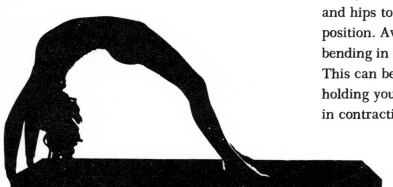

In a continuous motion,
raise and arch your spine,
evenly bending your shoulders
and hips to a back-bend
position. Avoid exaggerated
bending in the lower-back region.
This can be prevented by
holding your abdominal muscles
in contraction.

3. Equilibrium

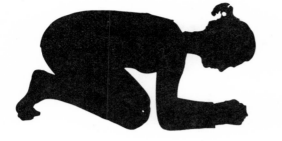

Assume a kneeling position
with elbows and hands
on the floor, one hand over
the other, palms up,
elbows and hands equidistant
from each other.

A. Place the top of your head
   inside your hands.

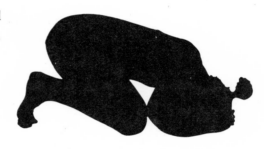

B. Pressing mostly on your elbows,
   slowly raise your hips.

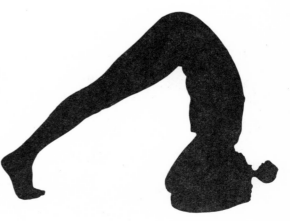

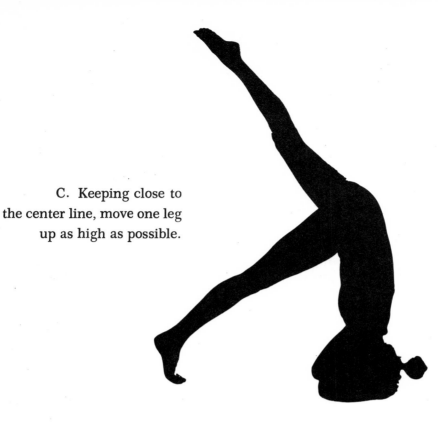

C. Keeping close to
the center line, move one leg
up as high as possible.

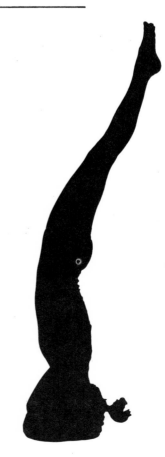

Then in a continuous motion,
slowly lifting the other leg to
join the first, gently arch
and control your balance,
using—above all
—your elbows and hands.
Your head is an extra support.
The headstand is a
stable balance like a tripod.
Nevertheless, to achieve
it, first gradually get used to
positions A, B, and C.
As a precaution, practice
facing a corner of the room,
hands about 1 foot from
the corner—or use a Nakbar
as a stopper, or,
even better, the strong arm
of a friend.

4. Strength

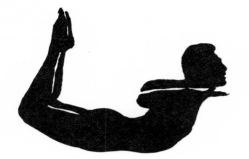

From lying in a prone position,
bend your arms and knees,
arching your back and trying to
bring your feet and elbows
as close together as possible.
Inhale.

Extend your arms and legs as high
as possible. Exhale.
Perform your quota to a slow
tempo—50 beats a minute,
with 2 beats for each movement.

---

5. Speed

Bending your left knee,
lunge back with your right leg,
hands on floor.

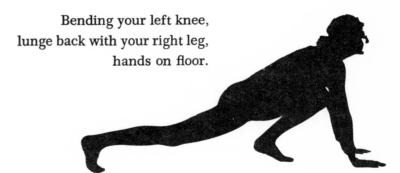

Then swiftly stand and swing
your right leg up.
Rapidly complete your quota,
then do the same exercise,
starting by lunging with your left leg.
Perform this as
quickly as you can.

6. Coordination

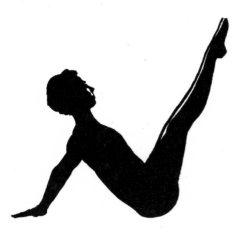

Balance on your hips,
legs up, arms outstretched.

Bend your right knee
and lower your right hand
to the floor, close to you on the
same line as your foot.

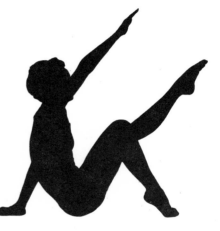

Pressing your right foot
and right hand against the floor,
in a lifting motion
pivot your body to the right.

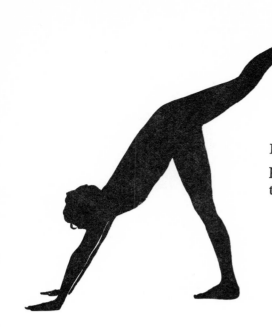

Raising your left leg high,
put your left hand on
the floor in line with your shoulder.

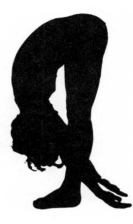

Moving your hips back,
bring your feet together, and
bending your body, swing your arms
back on each side of
your legs. Exhale deeply.

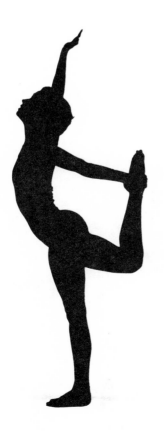

Rising up, swing the right
leg back, bend the knee, and try
to catch your right foot
with your left hand, at the same
time raising your right arm.
Inhale deeply. Repeat the same
sequence starting with
the left leg and the left arm.
Breathe normally except
where noted.

SPECIAL EXERCISES FOR WINTER

When the weather is cold, it is wise to warm up slowly to get your circulation going before attempting your daily exercise regime. You may begin while still in bed.

Follow a slow tempo of 50 beats a minute, with 2 beats for each motion.

1. Lie on your back,
   bend your right knee,
   and with your hands, hug
   it to your chest.
   Repeat with the other knee.

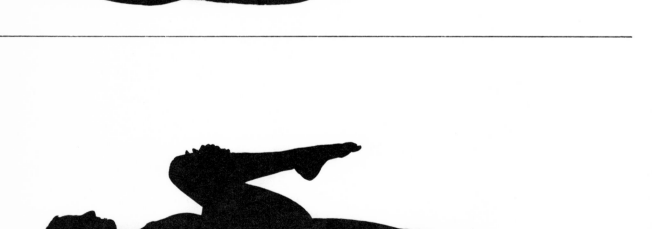

2. Still lying on your back, arms bent over your head and palms flat, simulate bicycle riding with your feet. Describe circles, forward and back, breathing deeply.

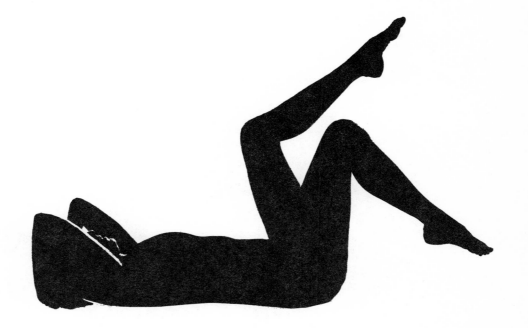

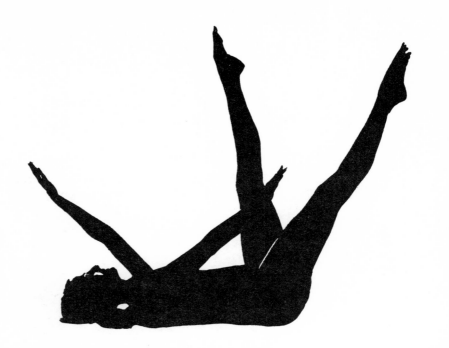

3. Lie on your back,
with arms and legs straight up.
Move your arms and legs
forward and back as
if you were walking on the ceiling
on all fours. Keep to a
regular tempo of 50 beats a minute.

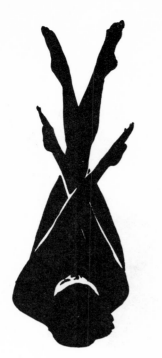

4. In the same position
   as the previous exercise,
   cross and recross
   your arms and legs sideways,
   alternating sides.
   Exhale while arms and legs are crossed.

5. In the same position,
   move your left leg to the left
   and both arms to the right.

Then move your right leg
to the right and both arms to
the left. Breathe deeply.
Tempo—50 beats a minute.

FOR SPRING

To adapt your body to an active outdoor life, you need to get your muscles ready to respond and, in particular, to train your legs for sports. The first need is to warm up your bending and extending muscles.

Maintain here a tempo of 40 beats a minute.

1. With your hands clasped behind your head, raise one knee high and try to touch it with your elbows. Exhale.

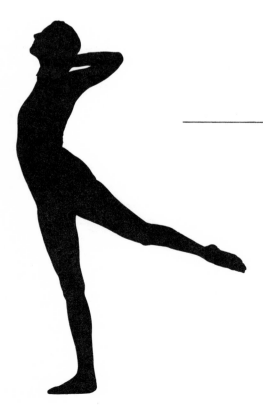

Then extend the same leg back, and at the same time bring your elbows up and arch your back. Inhale. Repeat the same exercise with the other leg.

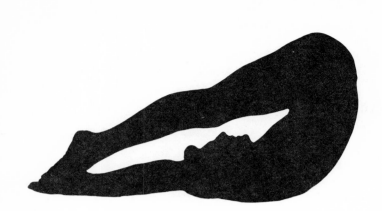

2. Lie on your back and
swing your legs over your head.

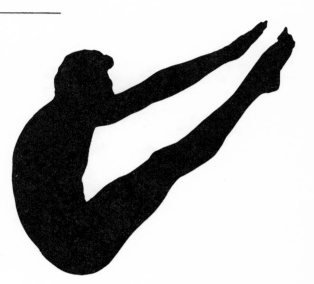

Then rock forward.

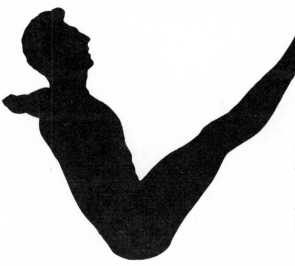

Balance on your hips,
legs up and arms stretched
out to the side.
Hold 10 to 30 seconds.
Breathe deeply.

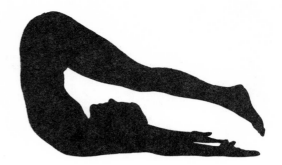

3. Lie on your back
with arms behind your head
and swing your legs
and hips over your head.
Exhale.

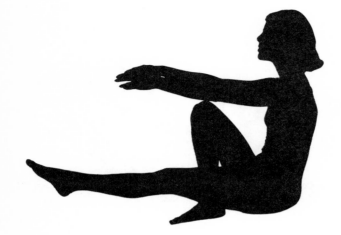

Then swing your arms and
legs forward, bending one knee
and keeping the other leg straight.

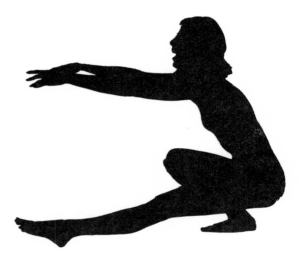

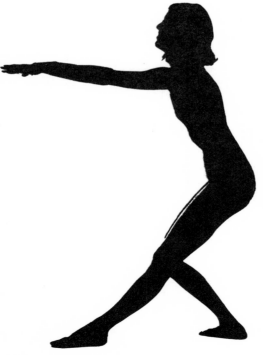

Pressing one foot and
the heel of the other leg down,
try to lift yourself to
a standing position.
Inhale standing up.
Repeat the exercise with
the other leg.

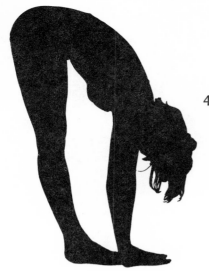

4. Starting from a standing position, perform the following movements in one continuous motion. Bend forward until you can put your hands on the floor. Exhale.

Then raise your body up, arch your back, and spread your arms sideways, while lifting one leg back and high. Inhale.

Swiftly move your leg forward, and bend your body until you can touch the toes. Exhale.

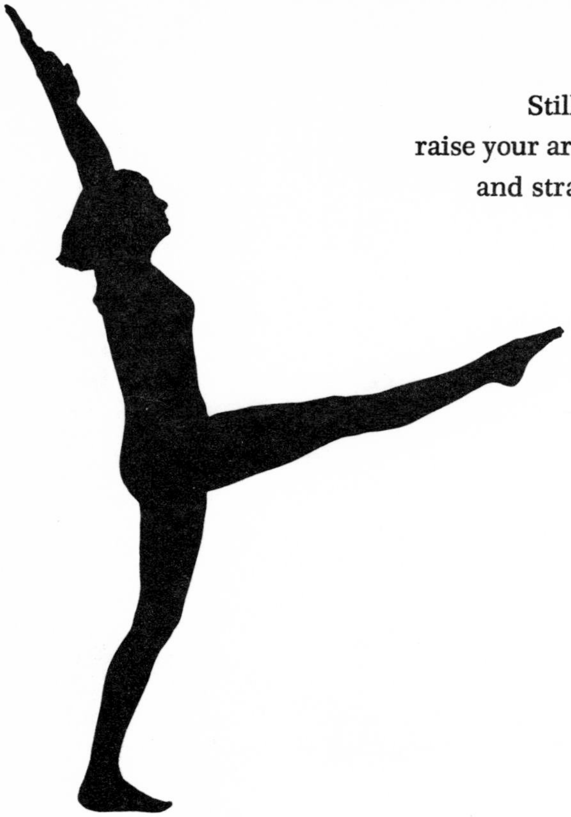

Still with your leg up,
raise your arms over your head
and straighten your body.
Inhale.

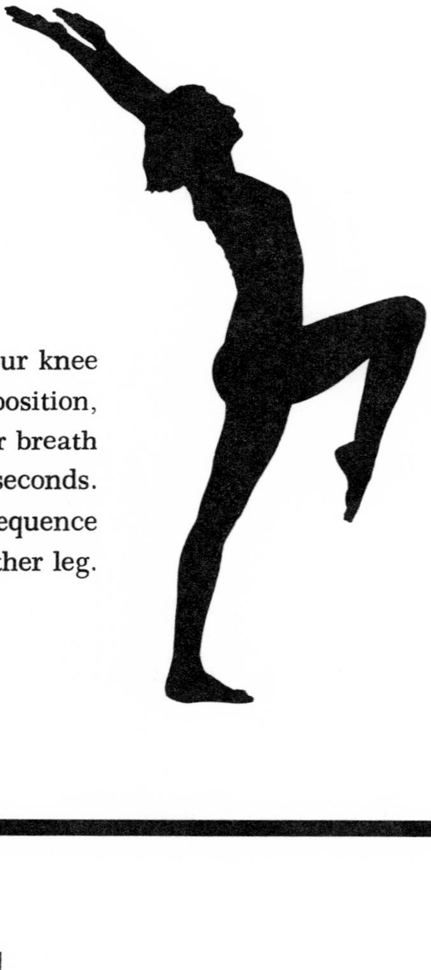

Bend your knee
and hold this position,
holding your breath
for several seconds.
Repeat the entire sequence
with the other leg.

Jumping

Find the most appropriate tempo, as it will depend on how high you jump.
Breathe regularly, exhaling and inhaling every 2 or 3 jumps.

To improve endurance you can repeat your jumps any comfortable number
of times.

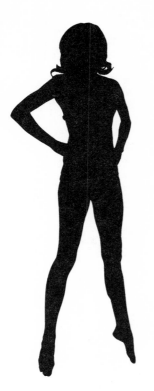

Try various jumps.
Start first with your feet apart
and then together,
touching the floor both when
feet are apart and
when together.

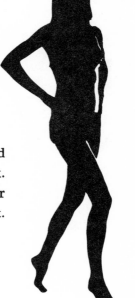

Jump with one foot forward
and one foot back.
Touch the floor
when feet are apart.

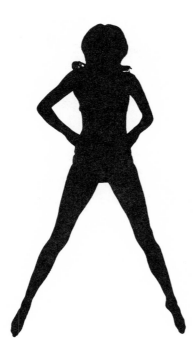

Jump with feet apart
and feet together, and this time
touch the floor
only when feet are together.

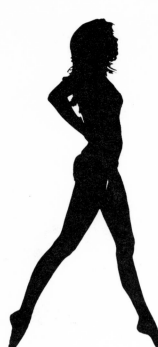

Jump with feet together
and then with one foot forward
and the other back,
and this time also touch
the floor only when
the feet are together.
Repeat, changing legs.

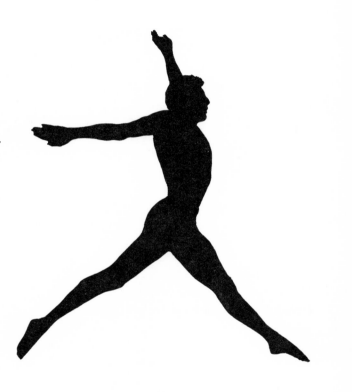

Leap into the air as high
as possible in a split position
as in the previous jump,
landing with feet together.

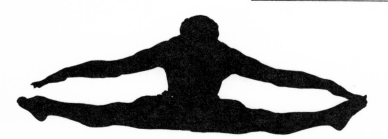

FOR SUMMER

When summer days draw near, practice your swimming strokes on land before plunging into the water.

1. Lying on a hassock or folded mat,
   perform the various swimming strokes
   as accurately as possible,
   breathing as you would if you were
   in the water (inhaling through your mouth,
   exhaling through your nose).
   Flutter your legs as you do the crawl,
   bending your elbow as your
   arm goes back, extending your arm
   on the forward stroke.
   Perform the strokes at various
   tempos and rhythms.

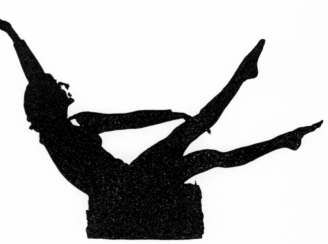

2. Balance on your hips and
   lower back and do the backstroke,
   fluttering your legs
   at the same time, breathing
   and tempo the same
   as in the first exercise.

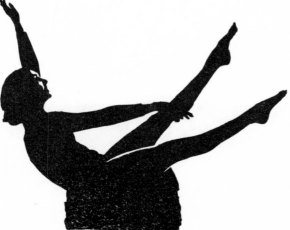

3. At home or (inconspicuously)
   on the beach, support your body
   on your forearms and feet
   for 10 to 30 seconds,
   breathing normally.

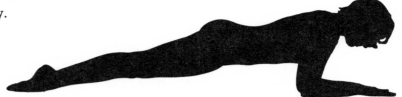

4. Fingers clasped behind
   your head, balance on your shoulders
   and heels while lifting
   your hips and body, and hold
   the position for 10 to 30 seconds,
   breathing normally.

5. Supported by your forearms
   and one foot, try to keep your body
   suspended for 6 seconds.
   Then repeat using the other foot.
   Breathe normally.

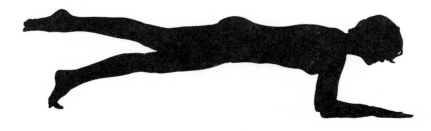

6. Lie on your stomach, arms bent,
   hands beside your shoulders.
   Push up until your arms
   are straight and arch your back.
   Curl your toes in.
   Perform slowly.

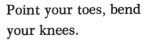

Point your toes, bend
your knees.

Then, gently arching your back,
bend your hips and knees
and try to reach your head with
your toes, breathing deeply.

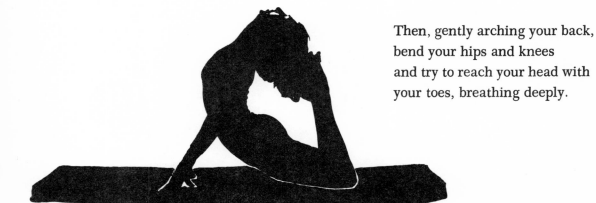

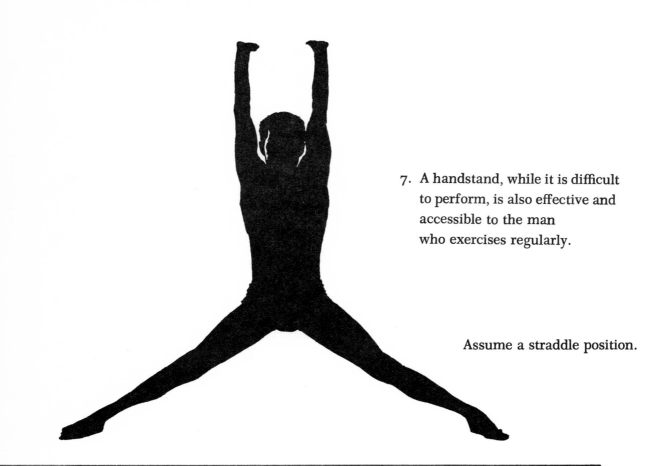

7. A handstand, while it is difficult
   to perform, is also effective and
   accessible to the man
   who exercises regularly.

   Assume a straddle position.

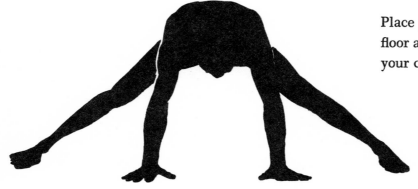

Place your hands on the
floor at shoulder width, under
your center of gravity.

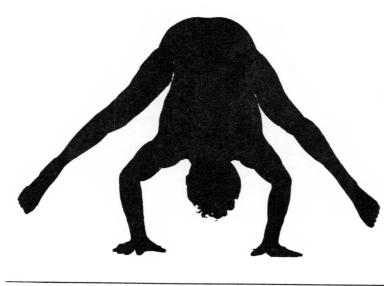

Slowly balancing on your hands,
raise your hips.

Gradually reach a handstand,
with legs wide apart.
Practice in sequence, close
to a wall, or with the help of a
friend. Try to breathe
deeply during the whole sequence.

FOR FALL

When the leaves turn and the air gets cooler, winter is near. Tune up your body for the ski season with pre-ski exercises.

1. Bend forward and move your arms to the right, bending your knees to the left. Keep your head down. Exhale.

Straightening up halfway, inhale, then move your arms to the left, knees to the right. Exhale. Perform in various tempos and intensities.

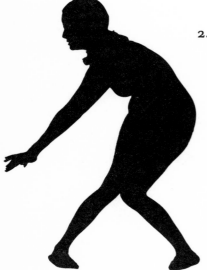

2. Stand with your legs apart, knees half-bent and held together. Bend your body slightly, holding your arms forward and down. Slowly twist your shoulders to the right, moving your hips to the left. Extending your right leg, exhale.

Shifting your body, inhale, then move your hips to the right, shoulders to the left and exhale. Perform in continuous slow motion.

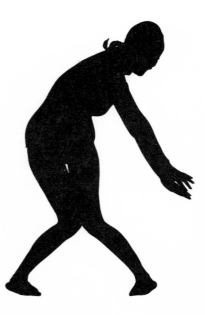

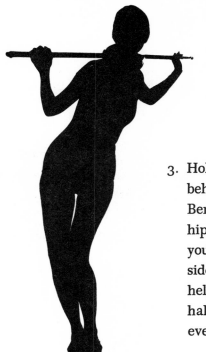

3. Hold a broom or a yardstick
   behind your neck, hands at the ends.
   Bending your knees,
   hips, and spine slightly, twist
   your body from side to
   side in a continuous waving motion,
   helped by shoulder and arm
   half-rotations. Exhale and inhale
   every 2 or 3 movements.

4. With your arms extended
   (use a broomstick to brace them),
   slightly flex your knees
   and bend your body from side
   to side, as in sliding
   against an imaginary wall,
   breathing every 2 or 3
   motions and gradually
   increasing tempo.

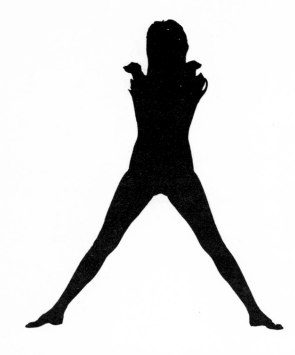

Standing with legs far apart,
arms forward, slowly
bend your right knee, keeping
your left leg straight,
then straighten up.
Repeat, bending the left knee.
(For beginners: Hold on
to a sturdy support.)

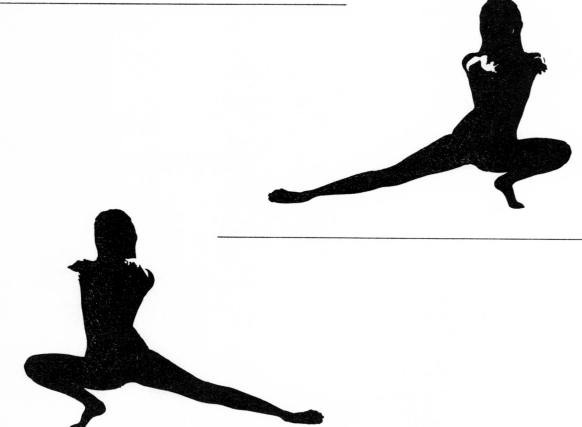

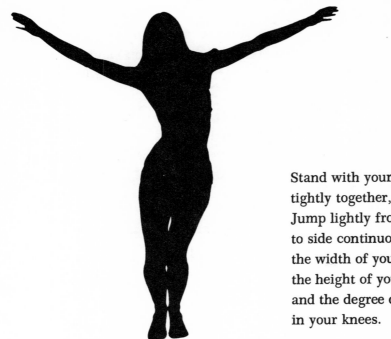

Stand with your feet
tightly together, arms outstretched.
Jump lightly from side
to side continuously varying
the width of your jumps,
the height of your elevation,
and the degree of bend
in your knees.

Try to maintain a comfortable
breathing. Continue the
exercise, making it comparable
to the time of descent on
your favorite ski slope.

PRENATAL EXERCISES

While it is very important to keep in good shape in ordinary circumstances, it is even more vital to do so when expecting a child. But you cannot usually initiate a regular fitness program at such a time, and you should not undertake special exercises without consulting your doctor.

Be sure that you wait two or three hours after you have eaten and that your bladder is empty. Wear loose clothing, and do nothing in a hurry. Take special care with your breathing and posture and cultivate an awareness of the muscles involved in each exercise. Relax between exercises to establish proper circulation.

Endurance

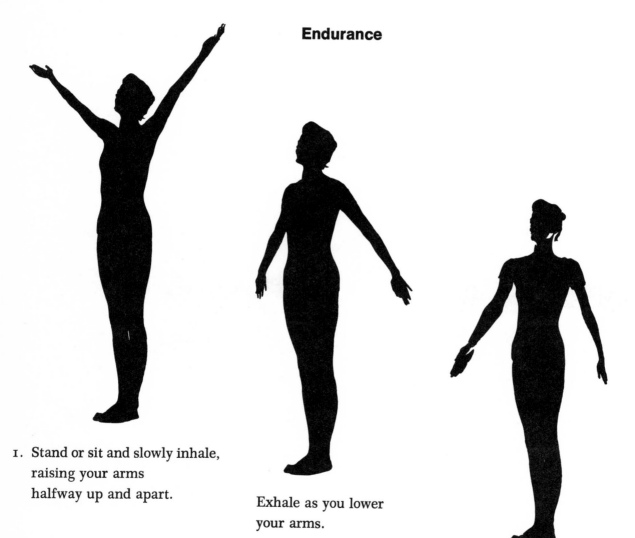

1. Stand or sit and slowly inhale, raising your arms halfway up and apart.

Exhale as you lower your arms.

Turn your body to the left. Repeat the entire sequence turning to the right.

2. Lie flat on your back,
   hands clasped behind your head,
   knees bent, feet together.
   Inhale.

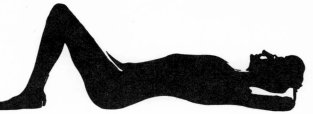

Contract your abdomen,
flatten your lower back against
the floor, and exhale.

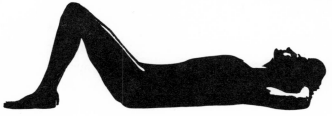

Suppleness

These exercises will help maintain your all-around flexibility and specifically will improve your pelvic mobility. Avoid overstretching, proceeding gradually.

1. Lie flat on your back,
   hands behind your head,
   knees bent and feet together.

Slowly spread your knees.

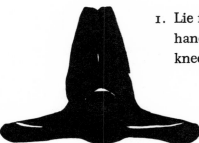

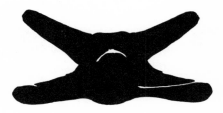

Hold this position for
a few seconds,
then extend your left leg.
Repeat from the beginning
using your right leg.

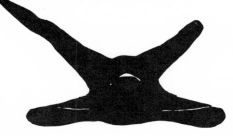

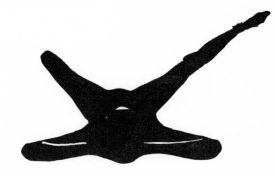

Breathe deeply and concentrate
on the muscles involved
in the exercise.
Proceed very slowly.

2. Support yourself on your
   hands and knees. Slowly extend
   your right leg to the side
   and up. Hold the position,
   breathe deeply, and
   return to kneeling position.

Repeat the exercise with
the left leg.

Equilibrium

Balancing exercises will help you control the slight change in your center
of gravity, and improve your sense of orientation.

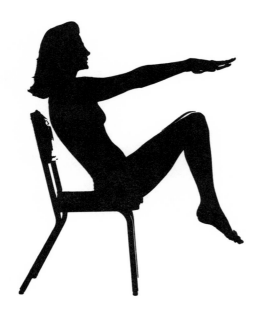

Sit on the edge of a chair
(not touching the back), raise your
feet off the floor, and try to
keep your balance.
Breathe deeply.
Balance 10 seconds at a time.

Strength

These exercises concentrate on the abdominal girdle, improve posture, strengthen hips and thighs. Avoid arching the lower back and synchronize your breathing to the exercise. Avoid overstraining.

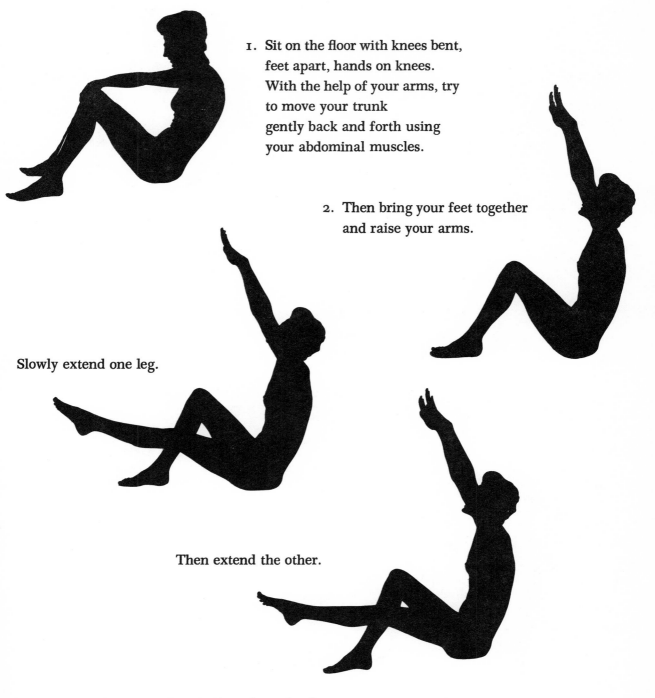

1. Sit on the floor with knees bent, feet apart, hands on knees. With the help of your arms, try to move your trunk gently back and forth using your abdominal muscles.

2. Then bring your feet together and raise your arms.

Slowly extend one leg.

Then extend the other.

Do all exercises slowly, breathing deeply.

Lie on your back,
knees bent, feet together,
hands behind your neck.

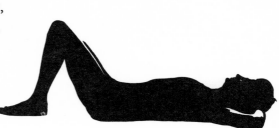

Hold your abdomen in,
contract your thighs, hips and
lower back, and slowly
lift your hips.

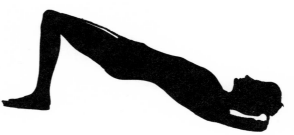

When you can do this exercise
easily, try straightening
one leg forward. Repeat the same
with the other leg.
Perform, concentrating on
every muscle involved.
Breathe deeply.

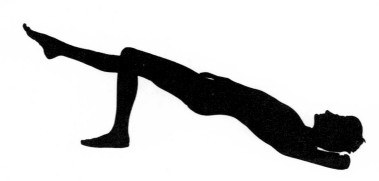

Speed

Avoid rapid exercising. If your doctor permits, continue with your favorite
sport but less competitively, concentrating on style rather than results.

Coordination

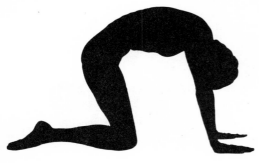

Support yourself
on your hands and knees.
Point your toes.

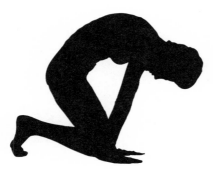

Rounding your back,
bring your hands close to
your knees, curl your toes in,
and exhale deeply.

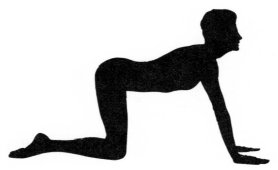

Then move your hands forward,
straighten your back,
raise your head and inhale.

Raise your left arm
in front of you and your right
leg back. Then start
again, ending with your
right arm in front,
your left leg back.

POSTNATAL EXERCISES

As soon as the doctor will permit (usually from ten days to four weeks), you can start an active, recuperative program for health, beauty, and vitality. Exercises will help you bring back your former figure (or even a better one), tighten up distended abdominal muscles, firm chest muscles, and improve posture. Wear as few clothes as possible (nothing tight) while you undertake the following exercises slowly.

Posture and Endurance

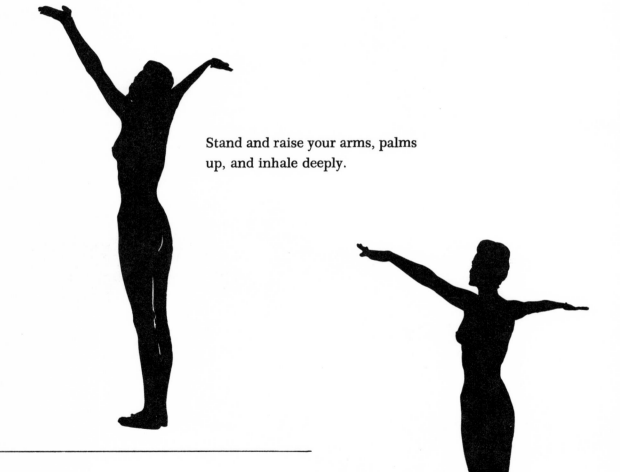

Stand and raise your arms, palms up, and inhale deeply.

Turn palms down and lower your arms to shoulder height, exhaling deeply.

To Firm the Abdominal Girdle

In the following exercises, exhale when you bend or contract your muscles, inhale when you relax them.

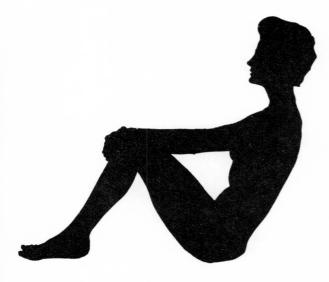

Sit on the floor, knees bent,
hands on knees.
Contract abdominal muscles.

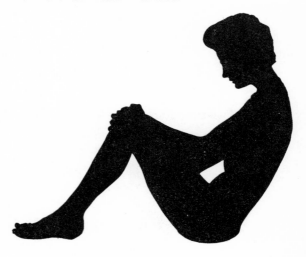

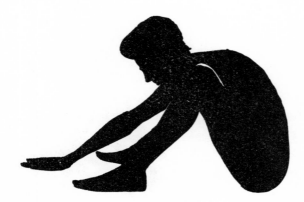

Feet apart, try to reach
in front of your feet
with your hands.

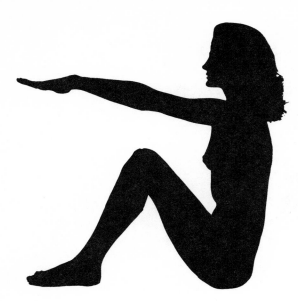

Sit on floor, knees bent,
arms in front at shoulder level.

Twisting your body,
try to reach far to the right.

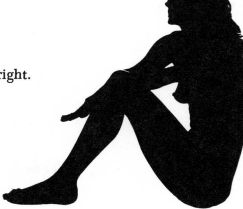

Then try to reach far to the left.

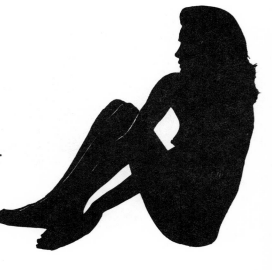

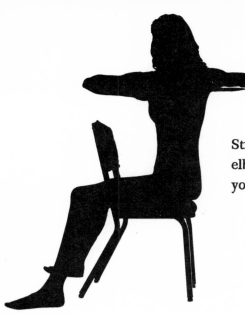

Straddling a chair, hands on chest,
elbows up, twist
your body to the right.

Then twist your body to the left.
When facing forward, inhale.
While turning, exhale.

Balance and Coordination

Sit on the edge of a chair and
balance on your hips.
Slowly bend one knee while extending
the other leg in front of you.

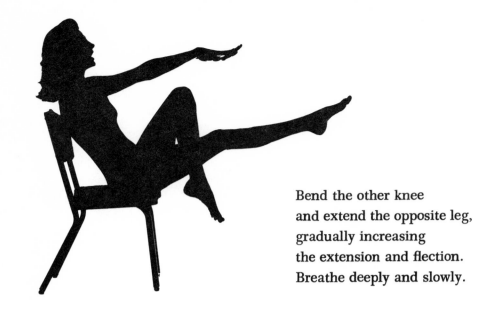

Bend the other knee
and extend the opposite leg,
gradually increasing
the extension and flection.
Breathe deeply and slowly.

After you are in better shape, add these exercises:

Posture and Endurance

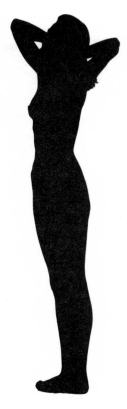

1. Stand with your hands
clasped behind your head and
slowly twist your body
from side to side.

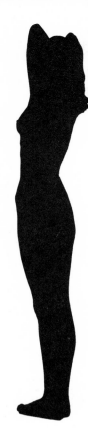

Then raise your elbows
high and hold the position
for 10 seconds, breathing deeply.

Pectoral Muscles

1. Lie on your back, knees bent
   and feet apart, arms up,
   fingers in and holding a pair
   of Nakbelles* or telephone books.

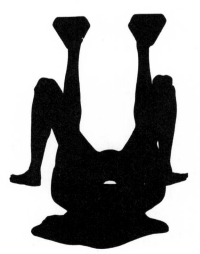

* See page 182.

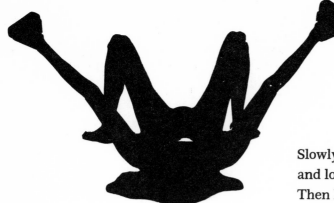

Slowly open your arms
and lower them close to the floor.
Then lift the weights up again.
Exhale when your arms are up,
inhale when your arms are down.

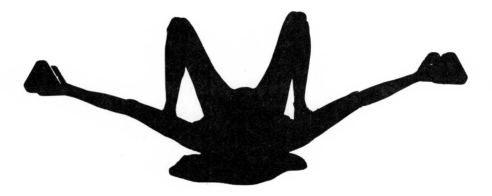

2. In the same position, arms up,
   this time hold the Nakbelles
   or telephone books
   with your palms facing forward.

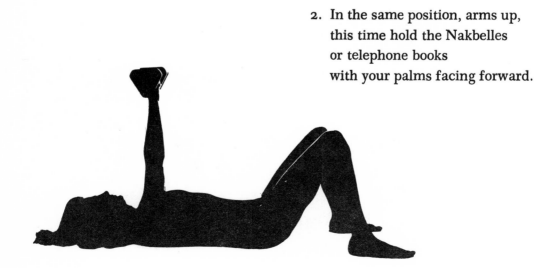

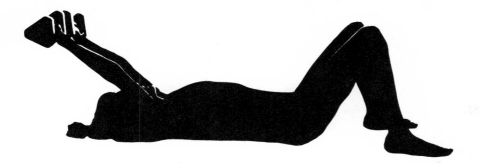

Slowly lower your arms
over your head. Inhale when
your arms are down,
exhale when they are up.
Keep your lower back flat on
the floor.

Waistline and Abdominal Girdle

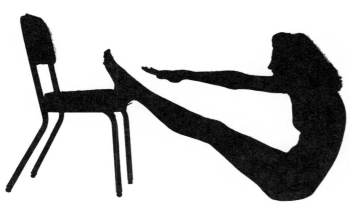

1. Sit on the floor, legs straight,
   feet on a chair, and arms in
   front of you. Try to reach your toes.

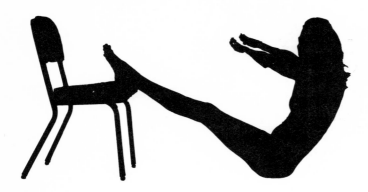

Twist to the right.

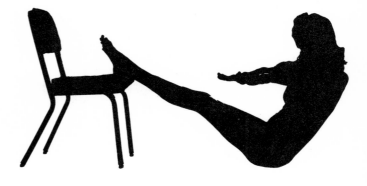

Then to the left.
Exhale when you contract,
inhale when you relax.

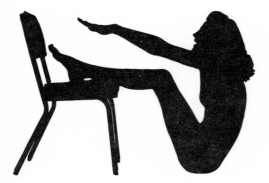

2. Sit on the floor, feet on
   a chair and knees half-bent, arms at
   shoulder level in front.
   Slowly try to touch your knees
   with your chest.

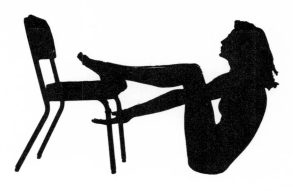

Do the same exercise
with your arms held down.

In the same position, twist to
the right and try to touch your
right knee with your left shoulder.

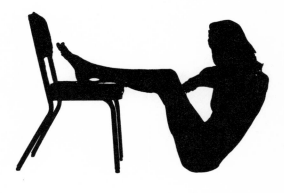

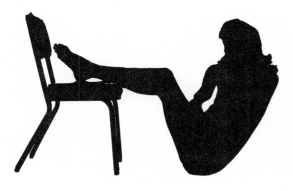

Twist to the left and try
to touch your left knee with your
right shoulder. Exhale
as you bend or twist.
Inhale as you straighten.

FITNESS FOR BEAUTY

That beauty is not skin deep is a true saying. Without inner health and fitness the expression in your eyes and in your entire body will not be radiant and glowing.

Every graceful gesture and every lithe movement add immeasurably to good looks. While a woman should avoid the kind of overdeveloped muscles that come from unwise or too strenuous exercise, to be beautiful she must keep her body supple and her flesh firm, and she must develop grace and coordination.

To maintain a radiant beauty, she should add the following exercises to her regular program:

1. Hands

Coordination of hand movements lead to graceful gestures.

Curl the fingers of one hand, and then gently turn your wrist in a circular motion while unfolding your fingers, as if they were the spokes of a fan you were opening.

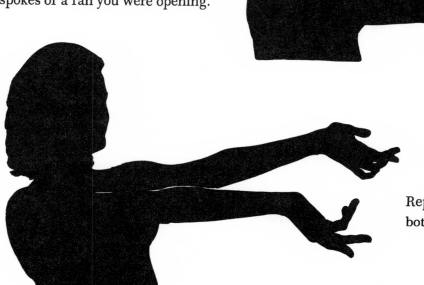

Repeat the exercise with both hands.

2. Complexion and Neck

A graceful neck improves the carriage of your head.

Recline, supporting your body on your elbows, knees bent, and head up.

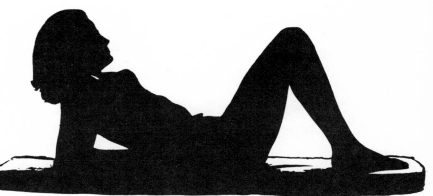

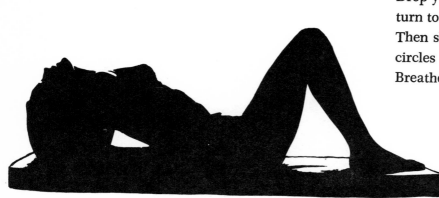

Drop your head back,
turn to the right, then to the left.
Then slowly describe
circles with your head.
Breathe deeply and slowly.

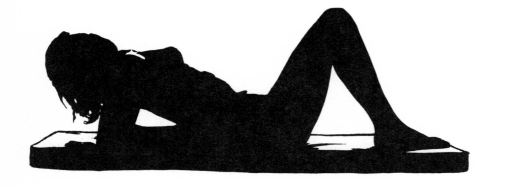

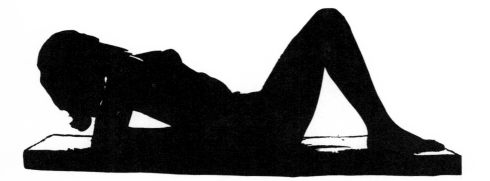

158

3. Bosom

A firm bosom is both fashionable and healthy.

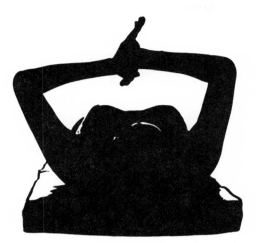

Lie on your back,
palms crossed and pressing
against each other
in front of your chest.

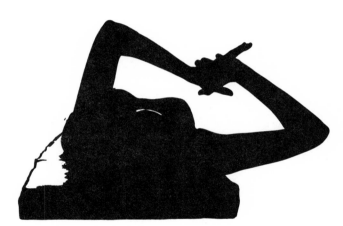

Still pressing one hand
against the other, slowly move
your arms to the right.

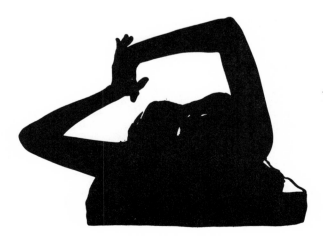

Move your arms to the left.
Breathe evenly.

From sitting on the floor
under a Nakbar, grasp the bar
with your hands,
contracting your chest.
Slowly raise your chest, lifting
your hips from the floor.

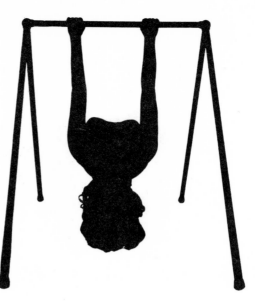

Arching your back,
let your head fall back loosely.
Close your eyes and
breathe deeply for a few seconds.

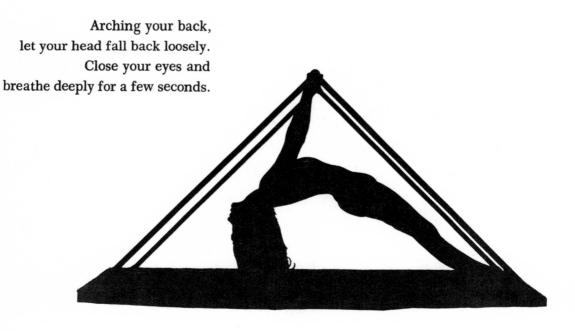

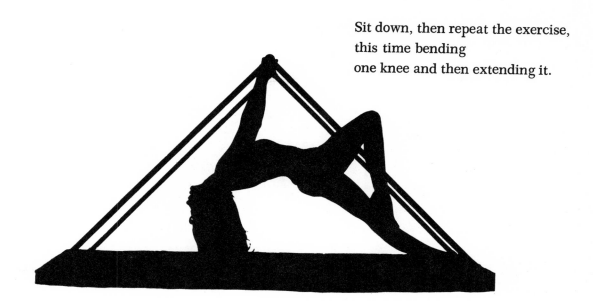

Sit down, then repeat the exercise,
this time bending
one knee and then extending it.

4. Hips and Thighs

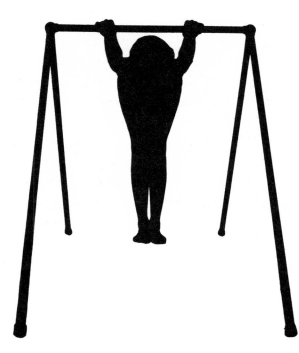

Stand with your hands
on a bureau drawer or Nakbar,
your arms straight and
shoulders down.

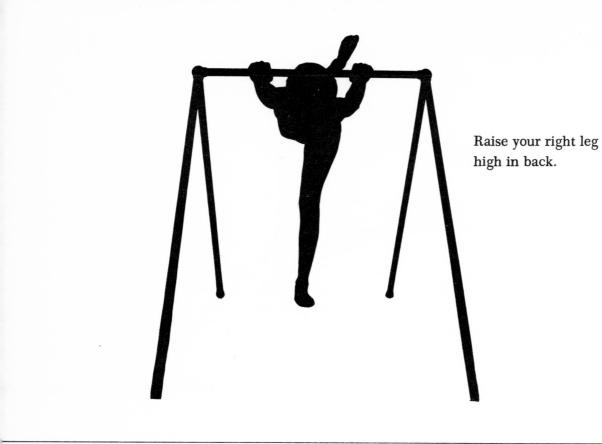

Raise your right leg
high in back.

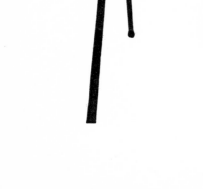

Move your right leg to
the side and try to lift it
to the height of the drawer or bar.
Then bring your leg to
the back and down. Repeat
with your left leg.
While moving your leg, keep
breathing slowly.

Kneel on hands and knees,
and lift and straighten your right
leg to the right.

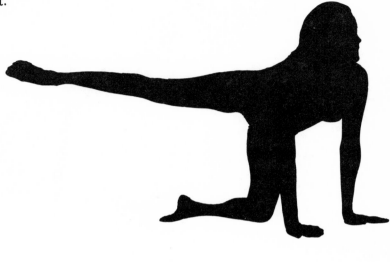

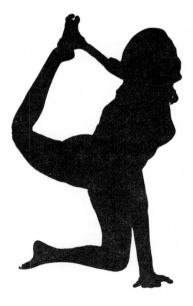

Then bring it to the back,
bend it, and try to grasp the foot
with your left hand.
Stretch gently while lifting
the foot high. Repeat
with the other leg and opposite hand.
Breathe evenly.

5. Feet

Feet are often confined and therefore lack proper circulation. They should be limber and expressive.

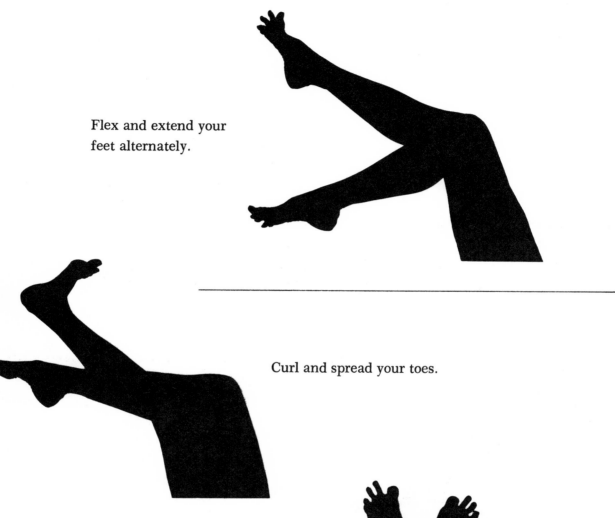

Flex and extend your feet alternately.

Curl and spread your toes.

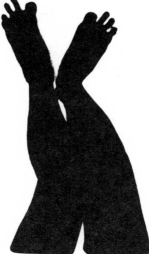

Keeping your knees and ankles together, spread your toes.

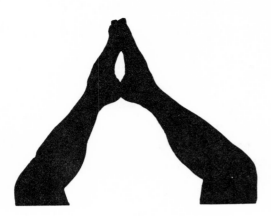

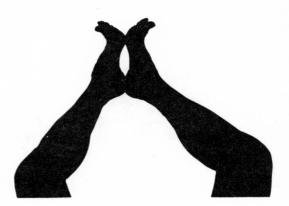

Then press the soles of
your feet together.

Spread your toes out.

6. Beauty Rest

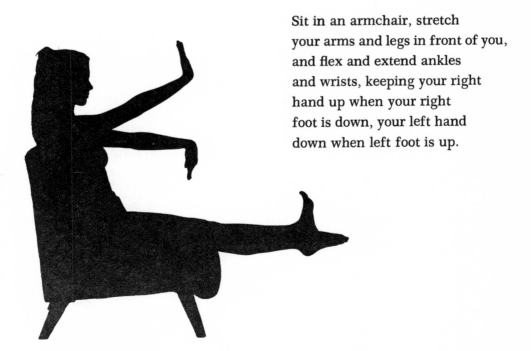

Sit in an armchair, stretch
your arms and legs in front of you,
and flex and extend ankles
and wrists, keeping your right
hand up when your right
foot is down, your left hand
down when left foot is up.

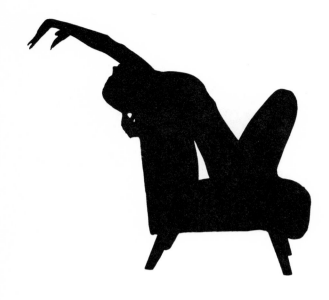

Still sitting in the chair,
bend your knees so that your heels
are close to your hips.
Then arch your back and stretch
your arms over your head
and breathe deeply.
Close your eyes and dream.

7. Beauty Stretch

Stand with your legs apart and
arms up over your head,
fingers clasped, palms turned up.
Stretch high and inhale.

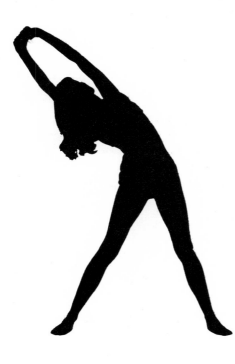

Keep stretching and slowly
bend to the right, sliding against
an imaginary wall. Exhale.
Stretch up again and inhale.

Continue the motion,
keep stretching, bend the body
to the left. Exhale.
Then to loosen up every muscle
of the body, bend
forward and relax a few seconds.

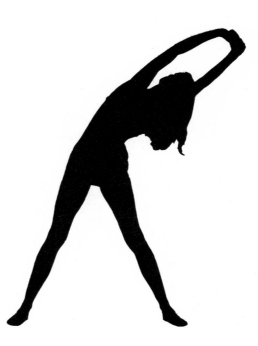

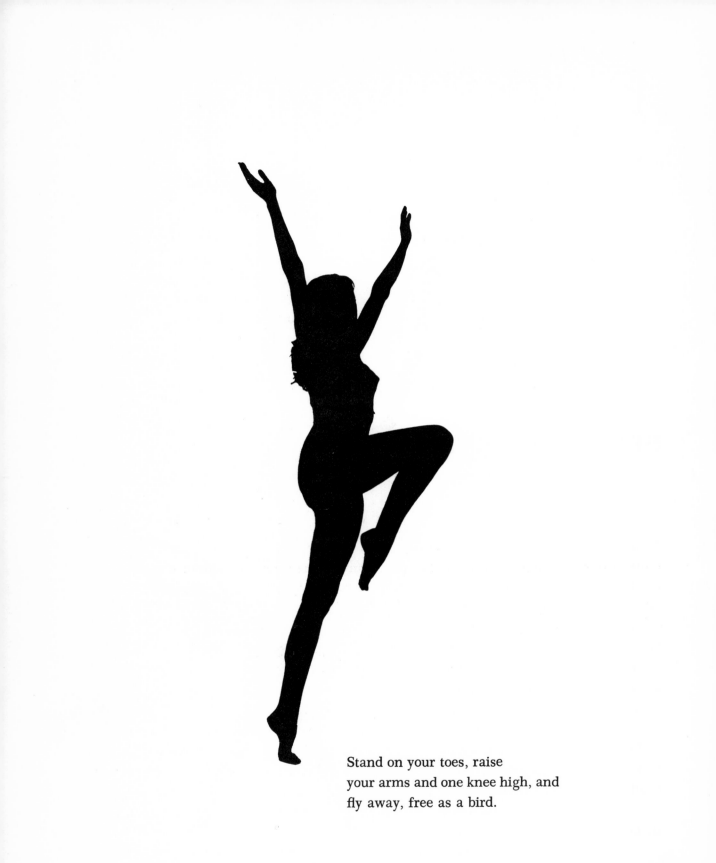

Stand on your toes, raise
your arms and one knee high, and
fly away, free as a bird.

FITNESS EXTRAS

In spite of modern conveniences, we are still often faced with problems that require dexterity or other physical factors. Once in a while we need endurance to catch the bus and not puff for half-an-hour afterward, or to climb a flight of stairs when we visit a friend. We need flexibility to bend over and tie a shoelace. We need equilibrium to stand on a stool to fix a curtain or to walk in a moving bus without losing our dignity. We need enough strength to open a jar or to lift the luggage to the top shelf, and we need the speed to dodge a careless driver or a slamming door. Our daily fitness program should allow us to face an emergency or a casual demand with ease.

Sports—outdoor, indoor, in water, in the air—help us maintain fitness and enjoy life. There is nothing more invigorating than to play a game of volley ball or tennis, or to dance, skate, ski, or swim. Many of these activities—if health permits—can be lifelong pursuits, carried on all year round.

Occasionally to enliven a friendly gathering or party, we may enjoy doing tricks or parlor games involving one or more physical factors.

Try a game of balance: Take an empty champagne bottle and place it on its side on the carpet. Sit on it long ways, legs straight in front of you, one leg over the other, only one heel touching the floor. In that position—balancing—try to write a message, read a paragraph, or simply unwrap a candy—naturally without touching the floor with your hands. The winner is the one who wrote the longest message or read the most.

Test your flexibility by standing back against the wall, heels, hips, and spine touching the wall. Put a pencil or a handkerchief on the floor near your toes, and without raising your heels or moving them from the wall, try to pick up the handkerchief or pencil with your fingers. Also there are games of strength you could try. For an opener, take a large bottle of soda. Holding it by the neck with one hand, slowly turn it in your fingers, always keeping the bottle vertical. Try to work your grip to the bottom of the bottle. Your fingers and forearm may rapidly feel cramped.

Or try a trick of mysterious muscular reaction. Ask someone to sit in a chair, deep and straight. Ask four volunteers to take up positions, one at each shoulder of the seated person and one at each knee. Have each one put his index fingers together, and have two of them place their touching fingers under the knees and the other two place their fingers under the armpits of the seated person, holding naturally just to get used to the position. Then try on the count of three to lift the seated person from the chair. Most probably nothing will happen. Release the holds and, one by one, have the volunteers put their hands on the top of the head of the sitting person—first everybody's right hand, then the left—pressing downward. Keep pressing for 30 seconds. At someone's command, all four persons release the pressure, quickly put index fingers together again, and place them in the previously tried positions. At the count of three again try to lift the seated person. Most probably—to your surprise—the person will feel like a feather and will be lifted up.

To test the real strength of a man's arm, try to lift a chair with one hand, holding the chair by the lower part of one leg; or as in the test we made earlier, stand on one leg and slowly descend and slowly rise; or try a one arm push-up or a one arm pull-up.

Add some table arm wrestling (Indian wrestling) or test speed by trying to pick a coin out of someone's open palm before he closes his hand. Or put four coins about 4 inches apart, starting on your open palm and continuing up the arm. With a swift arm motion, toss them up and try to catch them one after the other with a covering motion, before they reach the floor. If you don't succeed try it with three coins or maybe two, and work your speed up until you succeed.

As time goes by, your fitness program and your chosen sport or activity will guide you in balancing the energy cycles within your body. They will stimulate your physiological capacity and keep your mind alert, your body young.

Perseverance and regularity are the mother and father of success and achievement.

THE FACTS OF LIFE

Curing disease is a very lengthy and often unsuccessful process. Preventing disease is undoubtedly a much more encouraging method, but it requires active participation. To guide ourselves toward health and fitness, we must examine our living habits.

Whether you normally find the time for a run in the park with your Great Dane or the room for two desserts after each meal, you are observing certain customs. Our lives are so dominated by familiar patterns that we rarely look on them as "laws of habit" that we can keep, break, or change if we wish. And while most of us are proud of our good habits, we fail to identify the bad ones.

Your exercise dosage—while vital—isn't enough. Only when a physical regimen is coordinated with excellent and up-to-date health practices will you reap the highest rewards for your stretches and bends. It follows logically that the wrong habits will decrease the value of even the most perfect fitness program. As a doctor friend recently remarked, "To exercise without obeying the rules of fine health is like swallowing two pills: the first one makes you feel wonderful, but the second pill counteracts it." In other words, you are left right where you began.

WHAT AND HOW WE BREATHE

Breathing is the most automatic but most neglected of our body processes. Quite simply, we inhale the earth's atmosphere in order to obtain oxygen to keep us alive.

It goes without saying that we should consciously seek purer air to breathe —although this is often beyond our control. It is common knowledge that atmospheric air pollution is a serious threat to fitness—particularly to city dwellers.

I remember a cartoon that pictured a crowded room filled with smoke and alcoholic vapors. A bird cage suspended in the corner contained two suffocating canaries lying flat on their backs.

A fashion expert recently designed an "atmosphere suit" complete with an oxygen tank to provide an individual with his own supply of pure air. Besides worrying about this deadly threat, we can support legislation against it and seek purer air to breathe in our own immediate surroundings.

Breathing is a mechanical process accomplished by the muscles of the respiratory system. The diaphragm muscle contracts as you inhale, the chest expands, and the ribs rise slightly. This new space within you is filled with fresh, incoming air that is cleaned and warmed as it travels through the nasal cavities, enters the pharynx (along with your food), separates into the larynx, and proceeds to the lungs. Here the bloodstream absorbs the oxygen, exchanging it for used up carbon dioxide. Exhaling is a passive action in which the diaphragm relaxes, the ribs return to their former position, and this carbon dioxide is exhaled.

In active breathing this process takes place from 16 to 18 times a minute (though physical or mental stimulants such as running around the block or falling in love may accelerate the rate). It is a fascinating fact that as you breathe, every living cell in your body (including those of tissues, glands, bones) breathes also. When an emotion affects your respiration, it is actually transmitted immediately to the remotest parts of "you."

If you cannot always control what you inhale, improving the *way* you inhale has a positive effect upon your entire body.

Inhale through the nose, as if you were slowly sniffing a fragrant rose. This allows only the filtered, moistened, and properly warmed (or cooled) air to enter your nasal cavities and lungs. Allow the "muscles of active inspiration" to enlarge, and expand your chest as you breathe in.

Exhale through the mouth to expel all impure air without mixing this used air with the fresh, incoming supply. Allow the active muscles to return to their original positions.

Avoid holding the breath while engaged in activity. The more air you consume and the more you exercise the respiratory muscles, the greater the activity will benefit your body.

While active, wear clothing that provides adequate ventilation. Your pores are also breathing and need access to pure air.

UP IN SMOKE

People have been smoking for hundreds of years, it is true. But never before has there been such an emphasis on smoking and such a wide choice of smoking items—and such a plethora of reasons not to!

If I have gained a reputation for being an antismoking crusader, it is because I have observed the actual effects of smoking firsthand, in the studio. It is my firm belief that if everyone clearly understood what just one puff actually does to his system, no one would smoke. Remember, the first time anybody smokes a cigarette, his body's natural reactions are coughing, choking, watering eyes, and sometimes even nausea—something worth thinking about.

Those who have done research on the effects of smoking have no other interest than optimum human health. And despite the fiery debates and confusing statistics, sufficient correlations have been discovered to convince many people that smoking is a poison and obviously a risk to health. Every supposed "benefit" gained from smoking (relaxation, increased awareness, social ease, calming) can certainly be gained from less harmful substitutes.

Personal experience as well as experiments conducted with colleagues and students have shown conclusive results. One cigarette alone will affect heart response, blood pressure, breathing rhythm and regularity, and diminish physical faculties. In addition, a woman looks much more beautiful and a man more dignified when smoking does not mar their respective images.

There are many ways to stop smoking. A good idea is to experiment until you find a way that works for you. A journalist I know (who never used to be able to write a single word without lighting up first) began to record the time and place of every cigarette he smoked. He computed his average number of cigarettes per day and then very gradually decreased this number, still keeping a careful record.

Remember, it is advisable at least to moderate your smoking schedule if you can't immediately stop altogether. Make a special effort *not to smoke* at least a half-hour before exercising and a half-hour afterward. This precaution (which should not be too great a sacrifice) allows as much pure air as possible to get to the lungs, giving them a reserve supply of oxygen before your activity.

It also permits faster release of carbon dioxide and faster cleansing of the blood after exercising.

Many of my students find that an enjoyable fitness program helps them abandon cigarettes. "You stop *needing* to smoke when you begin to enjoy moving," an ex-heavy smoker informed me. And one encouraging note: When you give up smoking, your physical condition is restored to virtually that of a person who has never smoked at all.

NEVER SAY DIET

Just like any plant or other animal, we must eat to live. But social custom, routine, taste, pleasure, compulsion, nervousness, fear, and even boredom affect eating habits too. Most people know how important food is, but few actually know why.

Every part of you needs feeding: skin, bones, muscles, even hair and nails. What you feed yourself with is largely responsible for the way you feel. Different foods can make you tired, energetic, or even nauseous; they can also cause a host of more serious conditions, such as high blood pressure or hardening of the arteries.

Stomachs and metabolisms vary greatly. Each of us requires a different combination of foods, depending upon age, physical make-up, degree of activity, and life style. Eating habits vary: Some of us have numerous snacks "on the run," and others sit down to large regular meals. Some people find big breakfasts indigestible; others swear by them. A Mexican finds it hard to live without spices, and those raised on Italian cuisine have difficulty curbing their carbohydrates. There are confirmed vegetarians and "health food" devotees. And the variety of diets (for reducing and otherwise) is staggering. I have friends who might forget to eat at all if they didn't have important luncheon and dinner meetings scheduled. And we all know of individuals who seem to live from meal to meal.

Ideally, of course, a person should try to consume exactly what his body needs to be in its best state of health—and nothing more. But judging from the extraordinary number of dieters, this is not an easy goal to attain. There is one old cliché that is still true however: "We should eat to live and not live to eat." Henry the Eighth and his friends could perhaps afford to become totally immobilized for hours after devouring enormous feasts; but today's world belongs to the vigorous and the trim: sluggishness, an overfed appearance, and a lack of vitality are simply not in style.

What many of my students learn (and good eating habits are learned) is how to use their "appestat." This is a nonscientific term for a specific part of the brain (in the hypothalamus) that triggers a "stop eating" signal and thereby controls appetite. The study of human hunger control is still going on, but what we do know is that it takes self-knowledge, honesty, and discipline to train your appestat to behave.

After serious study of the "nutritional sciences" and after reading a wealth of material on the subject (as well as observing individual case histories over the years), I have come to the conclusion that nutrition is still basically a mystery to man. There are, however, basic "rules of the road"—or of the table— that we can easily learn to follow:

We need food for growth, maintenance, muscle repair, and proper functioning of all body systems and for production of energy to work.

We must eat the right amounts of the right foods to build and rebuild and repair body cells, protect against disease, and give us sufficient energy to function, to work, and to enjoy life.

We require different amounts of different foods in proportion to our size, age, weight, sex, and degree of physical expenditure.

The exact amount of each food necessary can be mathematically calculated and if functional requirements are normal, the intake of food can be precisely controlled. But due to the complexity of individual body chemistry, this theoretical precision is seldom achieved in reality. We should, however, be aware that our body needs:

1. Building and repair foods
2. Functional foods
3. Energy, fuel foods

These may be classified into six groups:

A. Milk and dairy products
B. Whole grain, cereals, and breads
C. Vegetables—leafy and root
D. Meats, fish, and fowl
E. Fruits—fresh and dried
F. Nuts and vegetable oils

If you can help it, don't be malnourished. I stress this quite often in lectures, particularly when talking to models or people who have to stay slim. In countries where food is scarce, to miss having the right foods is understandable but even where there is a great abundance of food available, a person can still miss eating enough of the right foods to become dangerously malnourished.

Avoid undernourishment—which simply means not eating sufficient quantities of food.

Avoid overnourishment—which simply means "too much" food.

Eating too quickly can impair your digestion and prevent your body from getting the full benefit of the food. Pleasant surroundings and a relaxed atmosphere are actually a boon to health. Well-prepared, appetizing-looking meals will give you the greatest pleasure. Time should be taken to chew each mouthful carefully; less food bulk can give you more nourishment this way.

Get sufficient rest after eating, as this aids the digestive processes.

Remember, improved nutrition automatically trains you to like better foods and decreases your body's need for unhealthy sweets and carbohydrates.

Never say diet and don't expect miracles. Think about eating sensibly rather than not eating. If you are making a special effort to reduce, avoid drastic measures. The best diets are those you are never conscious of because they permit food from all the nutritional groups. I have seen too many friends lose weight too quickly and then suffer the consequences, sometimes actual physical collapse. Skin becomes loose, muscles and organs lack the proper nutrition, and the entire body is put into a state of shock. (The same is true for rapid weight-gain plans as well.)

As a general body rule—whatever you want to change, do it slowly. Rome wasn't built—or unbuilt—in a day.

YOU ARE LARGELY WHAT YOU DRINK

Because the body is over two-thirds liquid, and a great deal of that is poured in, you are what you drink as much as what you eat. Fluids are expelled from the body through the processes of respiration, perspiration, and elimination. A good physical workout helps this process along; the body is thus freed of the harmful toxins that have collected. We are by nature able to maintain a comfortable equilibrium between dehydration and oversaturation. But there is a wide range of liquids to drink, and you should make the correct choices.

Very pure water (preferably from a natural spring rather than chemically treated) taken regularly is a perfect digestive aid and source of important minerals. Try to drink pure fruit juices (again in their natural state), milk occasionally (skim milk for reducers), and tea (good for relaxing you). As possible second choices there are coffee, fermented beverages, beer (rather fattening), and wine (which has beneficial digestion enzymes). Too much liquid during meals will delay digestion rather than help it. So will liquids that are too hot or too cold.

As for alcohol, it can mean enjoyment or destruction. Liquors are able to soothe nerves as well as stimulate quick energy. Predinner drinks have the effect of predisposing the system to food as well. But as you well know, dependence on alcohol—even to the slightest degree—can become an uncontrollable habit, dangerous to one's general health, career, and personal life.

One drink is often acceptable for the average physical system. While considered a depressant, it can also boost energy (just as a candy bar will) and has a pleasant calming effect. Several drinks can impair taste faculties, produce stomach spasms, and irritate the lining of the digestive tract. Sensations as well as thinking processes become considerably dulled.

As a side note: Straight drinks are less fattening than mixed drinks, but it is common knowledge that all alcohol is undietetic. Alcohol is a vitamin destroyer as well, robbing the body of valuable vitamin B.

To sum up: Drink occasionally for pleasure but never out of habit.

SLEEP

During sleep, our functions have a chance to slow down, and so do we. The brain clears itself of thoughts, and the muscles and joints relax. Sleep encourages the assimilation of the products of digestion, distributes oxygen to all parts of the body, rebuilds body cells, and prepares the individual for his waking existence.

The amount of sleep you need varies greatly in length and depth and depends largely upon your age and habits. The depth of your sleep changes from hour to hour. The most restful or deep sleep usually occurs after the first hour of slumber, and then slowly lessens until the time you awake. (Sleep may have a negative effect—weakening our systems—if we oversleep our normal quota).

Some of us are night people and function well with late schedules; others practically live by the sun. The best choice is a regular pattern and for this reason pilots live by their watches rather than by the sun and moon as they fly around the globe and mix time zones. Most people feel best with at least eight hours of sleep a night on the average.

Prolonged sleeplessness (insomia) affects the entire nervous system by causing irritability, loss of memory, possibly hallucinations, and body and mind fatigue. Relaxing exercises before retiring are the greatest boon to the problem sleeper I know of, while a few invigorating exercises can often replace the body's need for sleep, stimulating the circulation, and recharging the batteries. Well-timed catnaps are a wonderful habit. Even 10 minutes of sleep can allow you to awake with a refreshed view of life.

There is hardly any kind of fatigue that can't be overcome by either sleep or exercise. (By pulling to the side of the road and napping or engaging in some brief activity, you can avert the often tragic driving fatigue.)

BATHING IN NATURE

Man is healthiest when he is closest to nature. Even the world's most luxurious resorts and spas offer, as their greatest claims to fame, access to sun and waves, as well as natural springs and pure fresh air. Wind, rain, snow, and solar rays are our most valuable natural elements. The right exposure to these elements can help defend us against illness as well as provide a surprising amount of additional energy.

Overexposure, on the other hand, can disturb circulation, respiration, and nervous and glandular systems. A supposedly fashionable sun tan can seriously damage the skin unless it is acquired in moderate amounts. The body is equipped with a thermostat that allows us to enjoy varying temperatures of air and water. Steam baths or dry heat saunas, hot and cold showers, or sunbathing and skiing in the same afternoon are invigorating—internally as well as externally. Unreasonable extremes should be avoided, of course.

A relatively unexposed person can gradually adapt himself to heat, cold, and sunlight, thus tempering his body to the health-giving elements. But it is best to consult a physician before indulging in any revolutionary regimes, rigorous outdoor sports, or hydrotherapy.

JOGGING TO JUDO: A SIXOMETRIC ANALYSIS

Fortunately, statements that "proper exercise is as essential to survival as nutrition and rest" are finally being heeded. The ideal activity is one that assures you the most thorough physical exercise possible for the time and energy you expend. It should also be an activity that fits easily into your style of life—or else you will discover that you are just not getting around to it. A secretary I know decided to do a series of pre-ski exercises to get herself into shape. But she lost interest soon after she began because she "wasn't planning a ski trip anyway."

The form of exercise you choose should appeal to you personally. The disciplines followed in preparation for an Oriental priesthood or the rugged calisthenics of a military regiment, even in popularized form, are not necessarily appropriate to your life style. The best way to judge the exercise value of different sports or calisthenics is to analyze them according to the six factors explained in this book.

Jogging

Jogging is one of man's natural exercises. Yet this seemingly innocuous sport overstrains those who may not be accustomed to running or knee-bending. Joggers new to the sport should pay special heed to their body's own warning signals if they are not to overdo.

Yoga

The Hindu discipline of Yoga (Hatha Yoga is the one most commonly met) demands physical as well as spiritual concentration. The ritual makes use of several static body positions and the practice of deep breathing. Though Yoga exercises do relax and limber the body, they do not develop speed, keen reflexes, endurance, and strength.

Weight-lifting

This specific physical training is a limited form of activity that concentrates on muscular development and sometimes leads to overdevelopment. Weight-lifting does little to improve your endurance, suppleness, equilibrium, speed, and coordination. It helps build up strength, especially in men.

Ballet

Ballet is particularly useful to girls who wish to cultivate grace and enjoyment of movement. However the classical ballet steps and exercises lack certain factors both children and adults need to develop perfect fitness. Deep breathing is often neglected and the upper torso often underdeveloped, for ballet concentrates on the use of the legs and trunk. Endurance and strength as well as vital flexibility are not given sufficient attention.

Isometrics

Exercises with isometric contraction in which muscles without movement must work to oppose a force equal to or greater than their own—such as one hand pressing against the other—are helpful only as part of muscular training.

The static body positions are insufficient—a thorough program should, above all, include isotonic or active movement as well.

Sports

Many active sports both exercise and relax you, and most involve Sixometry or have Sixometric overtones. Tennis, for example, requires endurance, speed, balance, and coordination. A good tennis player however may easily lack true flexibility and strength.

Skating and skiing are both sports of balance and coordination. The control of the center of gravity is put to the test. Ice-skating and snow-skiing are healthy cold-weather activities that offer a good physical workout.

Roller-skating and water-skiing also give a beneficial effect as active sports.

Golf is hardly a true sport as it is not sufficiently active. Moreover mental tension on the links can actually increase one's stress and fatigue, while ideally your chosen sport should refresh you.

Swimming can be one of the most thoroughly Sixometric of sports, if one swims energetically. The suspension of your body in water allows great freedom of movement and the different strokes make use of most of the important muscles. Water sports are the perfect supplement to a personal Sixometric program.

Gymnastics

Having myself for many years practiced, studied, analyzed, and taught gymnastics, I realize that the special training can make unreasonable demands on the body. Certain feats involve extensive stretching of muscles and ligaments, which, in some instances, causes dislocations and overbends.

As for girls, any overstraining may lead to overdevelopment and even injury.

However, a judicious use of gymnastic apparatus can be very helpful in a fitness program. I have had exceptionally good results with parallel bars, rings, and trapeze set at various heights and carefully used, to help orient my students in support, suspension, and in space. Still, a gymnast rarely possesses the excellent posture and all-around fitness that you yourself will gain.

Acrobatics and tumbling are popular with youngsters but they become hazardous after adolescence and dangerous in adult life, unless you have been professionally trained and voluntarily accept the consequences.

Training for combat sports such as wrestling, karate, and judo is effective for self-discipline, confidence, and self-defense. But there is always a risk of injury, even in practice. Speed, strength (sometimes), and coordination are improved, but suppleness and general endurance may suffer.

Whatever sport you choose, you should enjoy it for maximum benefit. But you must also realize that no sport replaces a well-rounded fitness program.

LOVING

Loving is a marvelous exercise. Spontaneous or induced, it can be a gratifying experience. As with an active sport, or a dance, a 100-meter dash or a long-distance run, even a long walk, we have to be fit to totally enjoy and benefit from such exercise.

It is a great mistake to minimize the beneficial effects of healthy emotional and physical expressions, and it is just as unwise to ignore the demands imposed on our entire system by a profound demonstration of our mental and physical sentiments.

From its simplest form to the true art of loving, we may involve our total fitness. To make believe it is trivial to carefully study and understand the intricacies of such a natural habit and to overlook preparedness for it, are to ignore reality. An unhappy marriage or a broken relationship may be the result of such misapprehensions.

Physical fitness, as stated by medical scientists, "is the only way to augment sexual capacity by physiologic means."

Exercising beautifully enhances aesthetic feelings. Exercising soundly benefits our physiological potential. Exercising Sixometrically promotes the best within ourselves, and exercising with the right psychological approach leads to the most harmonious mental and physical state.

A marvelous link in the chain of happiness, loving enhances fitness. In return, one must be fit to enjoy the great feeling of well-being and satisfaction that comes from loving well.

HOME DEVICES

Nakbells and Nakbelles are specially designed devices to be used as additional weights. They are also used as handles for support and as stands.

A Nakmat is a practical, folding gym mat to be used in various thicknesses as a floor mat or hassock.

A Nakbar is a practical, folding suspension and support bar that allows all-around exercising in many positions.

All of these items are available at: Naks, 25 West 56th Street, New York, N.Y., 10019.